T0297866

Signal Detection for Medical Scientists

Signal Detection for Medical Scientists Likelihood Ratio Test-based Methodology

Ram Tiwari
Jyoti Zalkikar
Lan Huang

CRC Press
Taylor & Francis Group
Boca Raton London New York

CRC Press is an imprint of the
Taylor & Francis Group, an **informa** business
A CHAPMAN & HALL BOOK

First edition published 2021
by CRC Press
6000 Broken Sound Parkway NW, Suite 300, Boca Raton, FL 33487-2742

and by CRC Press
2 Park Square, Milton Park, Abingdon, Oxon, OX14 4RN

© 2021 Taylor & Francis Group, LLC

CRC Press is an imprint of Taylor & Francis Group, LLC

Reasonable efforts have been made to publish reliable data and information, but the author and publisher cannot assume responsibility for the validity of all materials or the consequences of their use. The authors and publishers have attempted to trace the copyright holders of all material reproduced in this publication and apologize to copyright holders if permission to publish in this form has not been obtained. If any copyright material has not been acknowledged please write and let us know so we may rectify in any future reprint.

Except as permitted under U.S. Copyright Law, no part of this book may be reprinted, reproduced, transmitted, or utilized in any form by any electronic, mechanical, or other means, now known or hereafter invented, including photocopying, microfilming, and recording, or in any information storage or retrieval system, without written permission from the publishers.

For permission to photocopy or use material electronically from this work, access www.copyright.com or contact the Copyright Clearance Center, Inc. (CCC), 222 Rosewood Drive, Danvers, MA 01923, 978-750-8400. For works that are not available on CCC please contact mpkbookspermissions@tandf.co.uk

Trademark notice: Product or corporate names may be trademarks or registered trademarks and are used only for identification and explanation without intent to infringe.

ISBN: 9780367201432 (hbk)
ISBN: 9781032016344 (pbk)
ISBN: 9780429259753 (ebk)

Typeset in CMR10 [font]
by KnowledgeWorks Global Ltd.

To our families, whose support and endorsement was absolutely necessary during this strenuous journey

"The author (D. Basu) holds firmly to the view that this contingent and cognitive universe of ours is in reality only finite and, therefore, discrete.

··· within the framework of a particular statistical model, the 'whole of the relevant information in the data' must be supposed to be summarised in the likelihood function generated by the data."

- D. Basu

in an article published in Sankhyā: The Indian Journal of Statistics, Series A, Vol.37, 1975

Contents

Preface

Data mining is a trans-disciplinary field of science in which a cross-cutting group of scientists use computer technologies, statistical algorithms, and artificial intelligence to find patterns or clustering of outcomes of interest in large databases. Data mining for signal detection plays an important role in surveillance for medical products including drugs, biologics, and devices. More recent research has revealed that different data mining tools have varied strengths and weaknesses depending on the statistical assumptions underlying their analytical approach.

Scientists have been investigating the use of data mining tools to identify drug-adverse event (AE) associations in large databases since 1998. Several algorithms have been described to sort and quantitatively evaluate the strength of AE signals. Disproportionate analysis methods have often been used to identify AE signals in drug safety databases containing spontaneous reports. These methodologies classify biological plausibility, number of cases, reporting rate, and health consequences to find important drug-AE associations. In 2011, the groundwork for the likelihood ratio test (LRT)-based methods was done in a research paper by Huang et al in volume 106 of the Journal of the American Statistical Association. The unique feature of this methodology when compared with the other data mining methods for safety exploration is that this method can control false positive signals at a pre-specified threshold and has high precision.

In the past decade, significant progress has been made in this analytical methodology leading to many publications. The prime motivation for undertaking the present task of book-writing stems from the need for a single source of the material published on LRT methodology. This book contains the development of the basic theory of LRT methodology using two simple statistical concepts, the likelihood principle and the design of a judicious Markov Chain use of Monte Carlo sampler technique to generate samples from an underlying model. This manuscript is an outgrowth of our lecture notes developed for a Food and Drug Administration (FDA)-India Office-sponsored one-week class taught at the All India Institute of Medical Sciences, New Delhi, India, followed by two other short courses offered at Bangalore and Mumbai, India, in 2011. Soon after these classes, several additional courses and webinars were designed and presented. In this book, the notations of the originating papers are preserved at the expense of redundancies so that the reader may find it easy to migrate to the original publications if needed. The objective of this monograph is to assemble and consolidate the material on various data mining approaches from statistical point of view both in Frequentist and Bayesian frameworks and on their applications that may have different features like continuous data, dichotomized count data, data with extra zeros, exposure information, longitudinal data, and data from multiple studies. We placed emphasis on LRT methodology, and we anticipate it would serve as a one-stop resource for future researchers of sophisticated, interactive, likelihood-based statistical methods. In that spirit, we have listed some applications such as medical device safety evaluation and site selection for inspection. This book uses the words "patients" and "subjects" interchangeably and has three parts, each containing several chapters.

The first part is devoted to providing background information about large data sources, introducing the concepts of signal detection, reviewing some data mining methods for safety signals, and likelihood-based inference. We provide the details of a simulation study for evaluation of performance characteristics of LRT methodology and of illustrations using FAERS data. We also discuss various extensions of the LRT method including double maximum LRT method for exploring safety signals of a drug within drug classes, modified LRT method and its relation to TreeScan methodology for detecting signals of multiple drugs/adverse events (AEs), and ZIP-LRT methods for handling data with large number of zeros. We also discuss other Bayesian data-mining methods including Simplified Bayes method, New IC method, and Hierarchical Bayes methods for signal detection.

The second part contains the definitions of drug exposure and multiple looks as well as the discussion of extensions of LRT methodology for multiple looks and multiple studies. Longitudinal LRT methods are presented with controlled false detection rate over multiple looks. We discuss how to analyze data with multiple studies or from different regions using pooled data or double maximum technique or weighted LRT technique to incorporate the variations from different studies. Modifications and applications to handle longitudinal clinical data is also presented.

The third part is devoted to presenting additional frameworks for use of LRT method (with modifications) in device safety signal detection with examples from Medical Device Reporting (MDR) data (post market device data) and clinical trial data, spatial cluster evaluation for device-AE pairs, normal-LRT methods for signals of continuous endpoints, and identification of site signals for inspection.

This book emphasizes computational aspect of LRT methodology and is suitable for first-time researchers and graduate students venturing into this interesting field. It should also appeal to academic researchers, faculty members, and graduate students in mathematics, statistics, biostatistics, data science, pharmacology, engineering, epidemiology, and public health. Therefore, this book is well suited for both research and teaching. It is our hope that this effort will serve the purpose it was intended for, namely, to make analytical techniques readily available via a comprehensive yet simple monograph.

For use of the LRT methodology, the zip file giving R codes is available at www.routledge.com/9780367201432.

We have had many fruitful discussions with many individuals concerning LRT method on signal detection. It gives us great pleasure to thank, in particular, Jianjin Xu, Zhihao (Howard) Yao, Yueqin Zhao, Ted Guo, Mary Jung, Rebecca Ward, Zhiheng Xu, Yu-yi Hsu, Jonathan Levine, Dan Zheng, Na Hu, and Tingting Hu who co-authored research papers with us on topics and tools covered in this book. We owe special thanks to Marianthi Markatuo, Robert Ball, Yuxin Ding, Estelle Russek-Cohen, Robert O'Neill, Lisa LaVange, Thomas Gross, Owen Faris, Daniel Canos, Jill Marion, Marc Buyse, Paul Schutte, Zhongjun Luo, and AbiAlbinus (Abi) D'Sa for their encouragement and support, and to Monika Deshpande for her editorial comments that led to improvements through-out this book. Finally, much of the research for writing this book has been supported by Food and Drug Administration.

Part I

LRT Methodology

1

Introduction

1.1 Background of Data Mining for Safety Signals

With greater technological advancements and medical innovations, post-market safety surveillance plays a critical role in ensuring public health. Companies manufacturing medical products evaluate the safety issues/signals of the medical products during product development and monitor them after the product is on the market upon approval. Consistent with the mission to protect and advance public health, FDA monitors the benefit-risk balance of medical products over their life cycle [50]. FDA's safety surveillance begins early in the product's life cycle as part of the review process that may lead up to FDA approval. Once the FDA approves a product, a risk-based post-marketing safety surveillance phase begins and continues for the life of the product [51].

According to FDA guidance for pharmacovigilance practices [13], safety signal refers to a concern about an excess of adverse events (AEs) compared to what would be expected to be associated with a product's use. A safety signal identified in the development and post-market surveillance may indicate a possible safety concern that needs further assessment. Such signal identification may be done using potential sources including large post-market databases such as FDA Adverse Event Reporting System (FAERS [4], formerly Adverse Event Reporting System (AERS)), registries, clinical trial databases, observational study databases, medical literature, etc.

The safety evaluation at the product development stage (such as Phase 2 or 3 clinical trials) is limited due to the relatively small number of patients/subjects enrolled and limited follow-up time. Clinical trials are usually powered for the primary efficacy endpoint(s), but not to study the safety endpoints. Collecting safety events, especially rare events, takes several years, which is not usually possible in clinical trials with a short (one- or two-years) follow-up. Therefore, some safety issues may not be identified during the development stage. It is essential for both companies and the FDA to continue monitoring the safety profile of medical products on the market in the intended patient population worldwide over extended time.

Large safety databases are usually obtained from spontaneous reporting system and some of those databases are described in the following section with details. Identifying safety signals using large databases is important for public health. Given the large number of drugs/devices on the market, monitoring safety of the medical products can be quite challenging for safety reviewers. Note that a single report submitted to the post-market database for an individual subject can result in many different drug-AE or device-AE combinations. The traditional methods of manually reviewing these individual reports are very cumbersome, time consuming, and cannot always detect the complex relationships between the drugs/devices and AE events in large databases.

Therefore, over the past 20 years, statistical methods have been developed and applied to large post-market safety databases. The process of using statistical methods to systematically analyze AE reports from large observational safety databases for determining the drug/device-AE combinations with unusually high disproportionate reporting rates (DRRs), using statistical methods, is called data mining or safety surveillance. Additional details of these methods are described in Chapter 2.

1.2 Post-market Safety Databases

Large post-market spontaneous surveillance databases include FAERS ([4]), the World Health Organization (WHO) Global Individual Case Safety Report (ICSR) database system (VigiBase [11]), EudraVigilance database (EU) [3], Manufacturer and User Facility Device Experience (MAUDE) administered by US FDA/CDRH [7], Vaccine Adverse Event System (VAERS, https://wonder.cdc.gov/vaers.html) database jointly managed by FDA and Centers for Disease Control and Prevention (CDC, US), Therapeutic Goods Administration (TGA, Australia) Database of Adverse Event Notifications (DAEN) [1], Medicines and Healthcare Products Regulatory Agency (MHRA, UK) database [9], Medical Device Safety Network (MEDSUN, US) database [8], National Electronic Injury Surveillance System (NEISS) database [10], and others.

The data from the spontaneous surveillance system usually contains limited information including the AE terms, possible reasons, dates, etc. There are also many registries for safety data collection constituting more information than the data from spontaneous system, such as a person-specific registry of medical histories, including use of medical products. The registries include Kaiser Permanente National Implant registries [6] for monitoring and evaluating the outcomes of surgical implants, National Cardiovascular Data Registry (NCDR, https://cvquality.acc.org/NCDR-Home) for helping hospitals and private practices measure and improve the quality of care they provide to the patients, Data Extraction and Longitudinal Trend Analysis (DELTA) Registry [2] for monitoring ongoing clinical datasets to detect emerging differences in safety or efficacy of medical devices, SEER (Surveillance, Epidemiology, and End Results) registries (https://seer.cancer.gov/registries/) for collecting information on cancer cases, and others listed by National Institute of Health (NIH) [5]. In the following, we provide some details of FAERS database (US), VAERS database (US), EudraVigilance database (EU), and FDA MAUDE database (US). The limitations of data from spontaneous reporting system are also discussed.

FAERS database

In 1968, FDA established the AERS database to monitor AEs and medication errors that might occur with marketed drugs. Data from AERS was moved to the FAERS for its launch on September, 2012 This database contains individual case safety reports (ICSRs) of AEs, which provide critical information to the FDA about ongoing product safety surveillance in the post-marketing period.

FDA primarily receives ICSRs from two sources: the regulated industry and the public. ICSRs from industry are sent to FDA on a mandatory basis by applicants/sponsors, licensed manufacturers, packers, distributors, and responsible persons subject to FDA's requirements for postmarketing safety reporting [51]. Members of the general public, such as health care providers (physicians, pharmacists, and nurses), patients, consumers, and family members, voluntarily report an AE either to the applicant or to the FDA [51]. If a manufacturer receives a report from the public such as a healthcare professional or consumer, the manufacturer is required to send the report to the FDA, as specified by regulations.

The FAERS database complies with the international safety reporting guidance (ICH E2B) issued by the International Conference on Harmonization (https://www.ich.org/). While adverse events from spontaneous reports are continually reported to FDA, some are submitted in periodic reports. Data in FAERS are made available quarterly online through Freedom of Information (FOI) Act (https://www.foia.gov/).

FAERS database includes demographic and administrative information; the initial report image ID number (if available); drug information; reaction information; patient outcome information; information on the source of the reports, and a "README" file containing a description of the reports. In FAERS, the Medical Dictionary for Regulatory Activities (MedDRA) is used to code events such as AEs, medication errors, and product quality issues.

The FAERS data are "cleaned" to reduce or remove duplicate reports and redundant drug nomenclature from the original submitted data. We do not discuss the "cleaning" protocols here, but note that in spite of pre-processing (cleaning), duplicate reporting may still markedly skew findings based on disproportionality analysis [70] limiting its use for data exploration.

MedDRA Structure

In developing and continuously maintaining MedDRA, the International Council for Harmonisation of Technical (ICH) Requirements for Pharmaceuticals for Human Use endeavors to facilitate the exchange of clinical information through a single standardized international medical terminology which can be used for regulatory communication and evaluation of data pertaining to

FIGURE 1.1
MedDRA hierarchy example

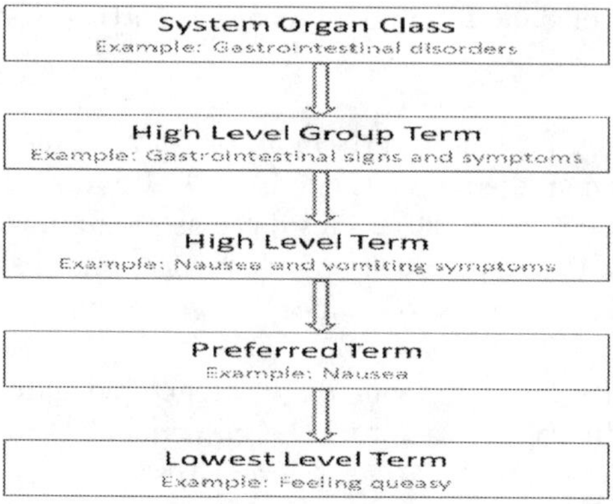

https://www.meddra.org/how-to-use/basics/hierarchy

medicinal products for human use (meddra.org/about-meddra/vision). As a result, MedDRA is designed for use in the registration, documentation, and safety monitoring of medicinal products through all phases of the development life cycle.

There are five levels to the MedDRA hierarchy (Figure 1.1), arranged from very specific to very general (https://www.meddra.org/). The most granular and specific level, called the "Lowest Level Terms" (LLTs), consists of more than 70,000 terms. The LLTs reflect how an observation might be reported in practice. They facilitate data entry and promote consistency by decreasing subjective choices. LLTs may also be used as the basis for auto-encoding. Since LLTs may be very specific, users can retrieve data at the most specific level of the terminology.

"Preferred Terms" (PTs), next in hierarchy, are distinct descriptors (single medical concept) for a symptom, sign, disease diagnosis, therapeutic indication, investigation, surgical or medical procedure, and medical social or family history characteristic. Each LLT is linked to only one PT. Each PT has at least one LLT (itself) as well as synonyms and lexical variants (e.g., abbreviations, different word order).

Related PTs are grouped together into "High Level Terms" (HLTs) based upon anatomy, pathology, physiology, etiology, or function. HLTs are in turn linked to "High Level Group Terms" (HLGTs), next in hierarchy. A HLGT is a superordinate descriptor for one or more HLTs.

Finally, HLGTs are grouped into "System Organ Classes" (SOCs), the highest level of hierarchy, which are groupings by etiology (e.g., infections and infestations), manifestation site (e.g., gastrointestinal disorders), or purpose (e.g., surgical and medical procedures). Additionally, SOCs also include issues pertaining to products and social circumstances.

VAERS database

Established in 1990, the Vaccine Adverse Event Reporting System (VAERS) (https://vaers.hhs.gov/) is an analogous database that underpins the national program jointly managed by the U.S. Centers for Disease Control and Prevention (CDC) and FDA to monitor the safety of vaccines licensed in the United States. VAERS accepts and analyzes reports of adverse events (possible side effects) after a person has received a vaccination. VAERS data are limited to vaccine AE reports received between 1990 and the most recent date for which data are available (https://vaers.hhs.gov/data.html).

The National Childhood Vaccine Injury Act (NCVIA) (42 U.S.C. 300aa-25) mandates that health care providers and vaccine manufacturers report certain specified vaccine events, as well as any event that is listed in the manufacturer's package insert as a contraindication to the vaccine (https://www.fda.gov/vaccines-blood-biologics/safety-availability-biologics/). In addition to health professionals and manufactures, anyone can report an adverse event to VAERS.

VAERS relies on individuals to send in reports of their experiences to CDC and FDA. VAERS is not designed to determine if a vaccine caused a health problem, but is especially useful for detecting unusual or unexpected patterns of adverse event reporting that might indicate a possible safety problem with a vaccine.

The information in VAERS data includes Person and Place (such as Age, Sex, State / Territory), Event Characteristics (such as Symptoms – classified with MedDRA), Vaccine Characteristics (such as Vaccine Products – vaccine type and name), Text fields from the VAERS form (such as AE Description), Date Characteristics (such as Year and month vaccinated, Year and month reported). Additional information about the VAERS data can be found at https://wonder.cdc.gov/wonder/help/vaers.html).

MAUDE and MDR

The MAUDE database houses reports of adverse events involving medical devices. It includes medical device reports submitted to the FDA (accessdata.fda.gov/scripts/cdrh/cfdocs/cfmaude/textsearch.cfm) by mandatory reporters (manufacturers, importers, and device user facilities) and voluntary reporters (health care professionals, patients, and consumers). It contains over four million medical device adverse events and product problem reports dating back to 1991 [44]. The information in the MAUDE data includes report source, AE (observed from patients), product problem such as device malfunctions or defects, event location, factors contributing to errors, actions taken to address the issues, and others.

Each year, FDA receives several hundred thousand of MDRs of suspected device-associated deaths, serious injuries, and device malfunctions [63]. FDA uses these MDRs to monitor device performance, detect potential device-related safety issues, and contribute to benefit-risk assessments of these products. Data are collected using two forms: the MEDWATCH form FDA 3500A (for use by user facilities, importers, distributors, and manufacturers) and the MEDWATCH form FDA 3500 (for use by healthcare professionals, consumers, and patients) (https://www.fda.gov/safety/medical-product-safety-information/medwatch-forms-fda-safety-reporting).

The coding system for outcomes in the MDR is based on the International Medical Device Regulators Forum (IMDRF) documents [63]. There are four types of terms/codes in IMDRF: Medical Device Problem terms/codes, Cause investigation terms/codes, Health Effects terms/codes (including Clinical Signs, Symptoms and Conditions terms/codes and Health Impact terms/codes), and Component terms/codes. Among the four types of terms, the Clinical Signs, Symptoms and Conditions terms/codes terms are closely aligned to a subset of MedDRA terms, through close collaboration between IMDRF and MedDRA [63]. From https://tools.meddra.org/wbb/, the clinical terms/codes in MDR data may be matched to a LLT or PT, and related higher level terms such as SOC can be obtained. Some clinical terms/codes may not have a matched LLT or PT, and one may consider them as single AE terms in addition to the LLT or PT terms for safety evaluation.

For mandatory reporting, manufacturers input patient problem code (health effects codes) and device problem codes (device problem, component, and cause investigation) directly into the MDR system. For voluntary reporting, FDA interprets narratives described in the MedWatch 3500A form and enters patient code and device codes into the MDR system. In this book, AE is used for the patient problem code.

EudraVigilance database

EudraVigilance [3, 14] (European database of suspect adverse drug reaction reports) is the European Union data processing network and management system for reporting and evaluation of suspected adverse drug reactions (ADRs). EudraVigilance system collects reports of suspected side effects. These reports are used for evaluating the benefits and risks of medicines during their development and monitoring their safety following their authorization in the European Economic Area (EEA). EudraVigilance has been in use since December 2001.

Patients, consumers, and healthcare professionals report suspected side effects to either the national medicines regulatory authority or the pharmaceutical company that holds the marketing authorization for the medicine. These reports (individual case safety reports (ICSR)) are then transmitted electronically to EudraVigilance. Pharmaceutical companies that hold the marketing authorization of a medicine, as well as medicines regulatory authorities in the EEA, are legally required to submit reports of suspected side effects to EudraVigilance. This includes reports received by the companies from healthcare professionals and patients.

The reports in EudraVigilance contain information about the patient, their relevant medical history, details about the side effect(s) suspected to be associated with the medicine(s), treatment, and the final outcome(s) of the side effect for the patient.

MedDRA is used to classify clinical information in EudraVigilance. Besides side effects (including diseases, diagnoses, signs, and symptoms), MedDRA supports the encoding of medical and social history, indications for use of the medicines, investigations, and physical examination findings.

Limitations of the large databases with spontaneous reporting

The strength of spontaneous reporting systems is that they cover all types of medical products used in any setting. Additionally, the reporting systems are built to obtain information specifically on potential adverse drug reactions. The data collection concentrates on variables relevant to this objective and directs reporters toward careful coding and communication of all aspects of an AE. The increase in systematic collection of ICSRs in large electronic databases has allowed the application of data mining and statistical techniques for the detection of safety signals.

Although databases from spontaneous reporting system are valuable sources of information on safety issues, they have limitations as the reports may not contain sufficient detail to properly evaluate an event ([13]), may not receive all adverse reports that occur with a product, and the reported event may not be related to the product. The information on drug/device exposure, indication, disease severity, and age, for each report is limited. Known or unknown external factors may influence the reporting rate and data quality due to the nature of the voluntary reporting. The incidence or prevalence of an event cannot be determined from this reporting system alone due to underreporting of events, inaccuracies in reports, lack of verification of the medical product causing the reported event, and lack of information about frequency of medical product use. There are missing and incomplete data that impacts the evaluation of the case. There may be over-reporting where medical products with well-known adverse event/product problems are more likely to be reported based on influence from media coverage – the so-called notoriety bias [119]. Therefore, the data from spontaneous reporting system may be incomplete, inaccurate, untimely, unverified, or biased.

Signals from the data mining procedure using the large post-market safety databases are typically used for hypothesis generation. It is difficulty to determine root causes for individual events conclusively due to limited information and no access to the actual medical product. Identification of a potential safety concern in large databases such as FAERS prompts, further evaluation which might include additional studies using other large databases, such as those available in the Sentinel System (https://www.fda.gov/safety/fdas-sentinel-initiative). Based on the evaluation of the potential safety concern, FDA may take regulatory action(s) to improve product safety and protect the public health, such as updating a product's labeling information, restricting the use of the medical products, communicating new safety information to the public, or, in rare cases, removing a product from the market.

1.3 openFDA for FAERS Database

openFDA is an Elasticsearch-based application programming interface (API) (https://open.fda.gov/apis/) that serves publicly available FDA data about nouns like drugs, devices, and foods. Each of these nouns has one or more categories, which serve unique data-such as data about recall enforcement reports, or about AEs. Every query to the API must go through one endpoint for one kind of data.

openFDA launched on June 2, 2014, at https://open.fda.gov. It features an open user community for sharing open source code, examples, and ideas. Medical device reports, enforcement reports, and drug AE reports have been available since September 2014, and any mention of a drug in those reports is automatically augmented.

Not all data in openFDA has been validated for clinical or production use. openFDA does not contain data with Personally Identifiable Information about patients or other sensitive information.

openFDA (https://open.fda.gov/data/) can be used to obtain FAERS data, MAUDE data, recall enterprise system (RES) data, structured product labeling (SPL) data, comprehensive NDC SPL (NSDE) data, and Tobacco Product Problem data. Of these, FAERS data and MAUDE data have been described in previous sections. Information about other databases can be found at https://open.fda.gov/data/.

2

Data Mining Methods for Signal Detection

Frequentist and Bayesian methods for safety surveillance can be used for analyzing large post-market safety data. The Frequentist methods include relative odds ratio (ROR) [124], proportional reporting ratio (PRR) [45], Chi-squared tests [61, 146, 147], and a recently developed likelihood ratio test (LRT)-based method [80] that controls the type-I error for multiple comparisons. The Bayesian methods for safety surveillance compare the posterior probability of joint occurrence of a drug-adverse event (AE) pair with its posterior probability under the assumption that there is no association between the drug and AE (i.e., the product of the marginal posterior probabilities of the occurrences of drug and AE). The methods include the Bayesian confidence propagating neural network (BCPNN) [22], Bayesian method based on a new Information Component [116], multi-item gamma Poisson shrinker (MGPS) [41, 133], and simplified Bayes (sB) [79], among others.

In the following sections, we primarily focus on the review of these common Frequentist and Bayesian data mining methods for the evaluation of safety signals in large post-market data including individual case reports obtained from spontaneous reporting systems (SRSs) such as the FDA adverse event reporting system (FAERS).

These statistical methods for safety surveillance, as discussed in Ref. [77], compare the reporting rate of a particular AE for a specific drug with that of the same event for all drugs. Alternatively, it may equivalently, compare the observed number of reports for the drug-AE combination with its expected number of reports, under the assumption that there is no association between the drug and AE. This can be viewed as comparing the conditional probability of occurrence of a particular AE for a specific drug (conditional on the occurrence of any AEs for that drug), with the marginal probability of that AE for all drugs. These methods do not involve the drug exposure-time information of the patient population exposed to a specific drug, but merely rely on the number of reports.

In addition to the above methods for evaluation of the safety issues for a fixed time, longitudinal surveillance methods ([32, 96, 102, 128]) include sequential methods for continually monitoring of an AE of interest for a specific drug. These methods are based on the case-counts for the AE or AEs of interest, and the patient exposure-time information from the drug, as the data on the AE(s) continue to accrue in real time. Comments on the development of the methods for active surveillance are included in discussion.

2.1 Review of Common Frequentist Methods

Usually large drug safety databases, such as FAERS data, include thousands of drugs and AEs, which can be presented in a data matrix with I rows (AEs) and J columns (drugs) as shown in Table 2.1. For each drug-AE combination (cell (i, j)) in the data matrix, the number of cases reported is defined as n_{ij}. Let $n_{i.}, n_{.j}$ be the marginal totals (i.e., the total number of reports) for the ith AE and j^{th} Drug; and let $n_{..}$ be the (grand) total number of reports. The $I \times J$ matrix can be collapsed into I, 2×2 tables (shown in Table 2.2). The cell counts are presented as (a, b, c, d).

TABLE 2.1
A large FAERS $I \times J$ table with event information.

	1	⋯	j	⋯	J	row total
1	n_{11}	⋯	n_{1j}	⋯	n_{1J}	$n_{1.}$
2	n_{21}	⋯	⋯	⋯	n_{2J}	$n_{2.}$
⋯	⋯	⋯	⋯	⋯	⋯	⋯
i	⋯	⋯	n_{ij}	⋯	n_{iJ}	$n_{i.}$
⋯	⋯	⋯	⋯	⋯	⋯	⋯
I	n_{I1}	⋯	n_{Ij}	⋯	n_{IJ}	$n_{I.}$
column total	$n_{.1}$	⋯	$n_{.j}$	⋯	$n_{.J}$	$n_{..}$ as grand total

TABLE 2.2
A 2×2 table and related notations.

	$Drug_j$			Other drugs: $Drug_{-j}$		
AE_i	n_{ij}	(a)	(p_{ij})	$(n_{i.} - n_{ij})$	(b)	$(p_{i.} - p_{ij})$
AE_{-i}	$(n_{.j} - n_{ij})$	(c)	$(p_{.j} - p_{ij})$	$(n_{..} - n_{i.} - n_{.j} + n_{ij})$	(d)	$(1 - p_{i.} - p_{.j} + p_{ij})$
Total	$n_{.j}$	$(a + c)$	$(p_{.j})$	$(n_{..} - n_{.j})$	$(b + d)$	$(1 - p_{.j})$

Let $AE_i, AE_{-i}, Drug_j, Drug_{-j}$ denote respectively the ith AE, $(-i)^{th}$ AE (all other AEs except i^{th} AE in the database), $j^{th} Drug, (-J)^{th} Drug$ (all other drugs except $j^{th} Drug$ in the database).

Let p_{ij} be the probability of the joint occurrence of AE_i and $Drug_j$; ie, let $p_{ij} = Pr(AE_i \cap Drug_j)$. Also, let $p_{i.} = Pr(AE_i)$, and $p_{.j} = Pr(Drug_j)$. Define the conditional probabilities as:

$$p_{j|i} = P(Drug_j|AE_i) = \frac{p_{ij}}{p_{i.}};$$
$$p_{-j|i} = P(Drug_{-j}|AE_i) = \frac{(p_{i.} - p_{ij})}{p_{i.}};$$
$$p_{j|-i} = P(Drug_j|AE_{-i}) = \frac{(p_{.j} - p_{ij})}{(1 - p_{i.})};$$
$$p_{-j|-i} = P(Drug_{-j}|AE_{-i}) = \frac{(1 - p_{i.} - p_{.j} + p_{ij})}{1 - p_{i.}};$$

The ith AE for j^{th} Drug is a signal if observed number of counts (reports) n_{ij} exceeds its expected number of counts E_{ij}, computed under the null hypothesis that there is no association between the ith AE and j^{th} Drug; that is, $n_{ij} \gg E_{ij}$, where $E_{ij} = n_{i.}n_{.j}/n_{..}$. Note that $n_{ij}/E_{ij} = \frac{n_{.j}/n_{i.}}{n_{.j}/n_{..}}$, which is the reporting rate of ith AE for j^{th} Drug over the reporting rate of all AEs for j^{th} Drug in database. If $n_{.j} \gg n_{ij}$ and $n_{..} \gg n_{i.}$ then $n_{.j}/n_{..}$ is approximately equal to $((n_{.j} - n_{ij})/(n_{..} - n_{i.})$, which is the reporting rate of AE_{-i}. Thus i^{th} AE is a signal for j^{th} Drug if the ratio, n_{ij}/E_{ij}, exceeds a threshold value such as 1. Usually a formal statistical approach is used to determine the threshold value, and may be taken as the lower limit of a 95% confidence interval for the reporting ratio (treated as a parameter of interest).

This section describes some common Frequentist methods for signal detection developed based on the 2 x 2 contingency table structure shown in Table 2.2.

2.1.1 Reporting odds ratio (ROR)

Reporting odds ratio (ROR) is defined as

$$ROR_{ij} = \frac{p_{j|i}/p_{j|-i}}{p_{-j|i} \times p_{-j|-i}} = \frac{p_{ij}(1 - p_{i.} - p_{.j} + p_{ij})}{(p_{i.} - p_{ij})(p_{.j} - p_{ij})}.$$

The estimate of ROR_{ij} is:

$$\widehat{ROR}_{ij} = \frac{n_{ij}/(n_{i.} - n_{ij})}{(n_{.j} - n_{ij})/(n_{..} - n_{i.} - n_{.j} + n_{ij})} = \frac{n_{ij}(n_{..} - n_{i.} - n_{.j} + n_{ij})}{(n_{i.} - n_{ij})(n_{.j} - n_{ij})}$$

Note that $\widehat{ROR}_{ij}$ is not defined (on the log scale) when the denominator is zero; that is, when either $n_{i.} - n_{ij} = 0$ or $n_{.j} - n_{ij} = 0$. Using the delta method,

$$log(\widehat{ROR}_{ij}) \sim N(log(ROR_{ij}), \sigma^2_{log(ROR)_{ij}}),$$
$$\hat{\sigma}^2_{log(ROR)_{ij}} \approx \frac{1}{n_{ij}} + \frac{1}{(n_{i.} - n_{ij})} + \frac{1}{(n_{.j} - n_{ij})} + \frac{1}{(n_{..} - n_{i.} - n_{.j} + n_{ij})}.$$

The approximate $100(1-\alpha)\%$ confidence interval (CI) for $\widehat{ROR}_{ij}$ is given by:

$$CI_{ROR_{ij},100(1-\alpha)\%} = \exp\left(log(\widehat{ROR}_{ij}) \pm z_{1-\alpha/2}\sqrt{\hat{\sigma}^2_{log(ROR)_{ij}}}\right),$$

where $z_{1-\alpha/2} = \Phi(1-\alpha/2)$ and Φ is the cumulative distribution function of the standard normal distribution. Here and throughout, unless explicitly specified, the notation, $log(x)$ or $ln(x)$ is meant to be the natural logarithm function of x.

For fixed pair $(AE_i, Drug_j)$, consider testing the null hypothesis that $H_0 : ROR_{ij} = 1$; that is, $H_0 : p_{ij} = p_{i.} \times p_{.j}$ versus the (one-sided) alternative hypothesis that $H_a : ROR_{ij} > 1$; that is $H_a : p_{ij} > p_{i.} \times p_{.j}$ at a specified two-sided level of significance, $\alpha = 0.05$. If the lower bound of this confidence interval $CI_{ROR_{ij},95\%}$ is greater than 1, the ith AE can be interpreted as a signal of disproportionate rate (SDR) for the jth Drug.

2.1.2 Proportional reporting ratio

Given the above 2×2 contingency table of the reports on the ith AE and j^{th} Drug, the proportional reporting ratio (PRR) is defined as

$$PRR_{ij} = \frac{p_{j|i}}{p_{j|-i}} = \frac{p_{ij}/p_{i.}}{(p_{.j} - p_{ij})/(1-p_{i.})}.$$

PRR can be interpreted as ratio of the proportion of the number of reports of the ith AE for j^{th} Drug to the corresponding proportion of reports of all other AEs for the jth Drug in the whole database.

Its estimate is given by

$$\widehat{PRR}_{ij} = \frac{n_{ij}/n_{i.}}{(n_{.j} - n_{ij})/(n_{..} - n_{i.})} = \frac{n_{ij}(n_{..} - n_{i.})}{n_{i.}(n_{.j} - n_{ij})}$$

This measure is the relative reporting rate of ith AE vs. other AEs for j^{th} Drug.

Note that if $n_{i.} - n_{ij} \approx n_{i.}$ and $n_{..} - n_{i.} - n_{.j} + n_{ij}) \approx n_{..} - n_{i.}$, then $\widehat{ROR}_{ij} \approx \widehat{PRR}_{ij}$. Also, $log(\widehat{PRR}_{ij}) \sim N(log(PRR_{ij}), \sigma^2_{log(PRR)_{ij}})$, where $\sigma^2_{log(PRR)_{ij}} \approx \frac{1}{n_{ij}} - \frac{1}{n_{i.}} + \frac{1}{n_{.j}-n_{ij}} - \frac{1}{n_{..}-n_{i.}}$.

An approximate 95% CI for PRR_{ij} with $\alpha = 0.05$ is given by

$$CI_{PRR_{ij},100(1-\alpha)\%} = exp\left(log(\widehat{PRR}_{ij}) \pm z_{1-\alpha/2}\sqrt{\hat{\sigma}^2_{log(PRR)_{ij}}}\right)$$
$$= exp\left[log(\widehat{PRR}_{ij}) \pm 1.96\sqrt{1/n_{ij} - 1/n_{i.} + 1/(n_{.j} - n_{ij}) - 1/(n_{..} - n_{i.})}\right].$$

The decision making criterion for i^{th} AE to be a SDR is same as that of ROR [67].

There have been suggestions [45] to restrict $n_{ij} > 3$ or more cases, and to raise the threshold from 1 to 2 in order to reduce the false positive signals for PRR and ROR methods.

2.1.3 Information component

The information component (IC) is defined based on relative reporting rate (RR), which is $RR_{ij} = \frac{p_{i|j}}{p_{i.}} = \frac{p_{ij}}{p_{i.} \times p_{.j}}$. The estimate of RR_{ij} is

$$\widehat{RR}_{ij} = \frac{n_{ij}/n_{i.}}{n_{.j}/n_{..}} = \frac{n_{ij}}{(n_{i.}n_{.j})/n_{..}} = \frac{n_{ij}}{E_{ij}},$$

where $E_{ij} = \frac{n_{i.} \times n_{.j}}{n_{..}}$, is the expected number of reports for the cell $(AE_i, Drug_j)$, under the null hypothesis $H_{ij} : p_{ij} = p_{i.} \times p_{.j}$. Here the RR is the rate for i^{th} AE over the rate for all AEs (for a fixed j^{th} Drug). Another way to define RR is to use the rate for all AEs excluding i^{th} AE (row) in the denominator; that is, let

$$\widehat{RR}^*_{ij} = \frac{n_{ij}/n_{i.}}{(n_{.j} - n_{ij})/(n_{..} - n_{i.})}.$$

Note that $\widehat{RR}^*_{ij}$ is close to $\widehat{RR}_{ij}$ when $n_{.j}$ and $n_{..}$ are large compared to n_{ij} and $n_{i.}$, respectively.

The IC is defined as

$$IC_{ij} = log_2(RR_{ij}) = log_2(\frac{p_{ij}}{p_{i.} \times p_{.j}}) = \frac{log(RR_{ij})}{ln(2)}$$

An estimate of IC_{ij} is

$$\widehat{IC}_{ij} = log_2(\frac{\hat{p}_{ij}}{\hat{p}_{i.} \times \hat{p}_{.j}}) = log_2(\frac{n_{ij}}{n_{i.} \times n_{.j}/n_{..}}) = log_2(\frac{n_{ij}}{E_{ij}}),$$

provided that it is defined; that is, $n_{ij} > 0, n_{i.} > 0, n_{.j} > 0$. An estimate of the variance of $\widehat{IC}_{ij}$ is given by

$$\hat{\sigma}^2_{\widehat{IC}_{ij}} \approx \frac{1}{(log2)^2}\left[\frac{1}{n_{ij}} + \frac{1}{n_{i.}} + \frac{1}{n_{.j}}\right]$$

A 95% confidence interval (CI) for IC can be obtained with normality assumption. If the lower bound of 95% CI of IC is greater than 0, the ith AE can be interpreted as a signal of disproportionate rate (SDR) for the jth Drug.

2.1.4 Chi-squared test

A Chi-squared test of independence $H_0 : p_{ij} = p_{i.} \times p_{.j}$ between $Drug_j$ and AE_i is given by

$$\begin{aligned}\chi^2_{ij} &= \sum (O - E)^2/E \\ &= \frac{(O_{11} - E_{11})^2}{E_{11}} + \frac{(O_{21} - E_{21})^2}{E_{21}} + \frac{(O_{12} - E_{12})^2}{E_{12}} + \frac{(O_{22} - E_{22})^2}{E_{22}},\end{aligned}$$

where O denotes the observed frequency and E denotes the expected frequency for each cells $(1,1), (2,1), (1,2)$, and $(2,2)$ in i^{th} 2×2 table (with fixed j) shown in Table 2.2, respectively.

Under the null hypothesis of independence (H_0), the statistic

$$\chi^2_{ij} = \frac{(a+b+c+d)(ad-ac)^2}{(a+b)(a+c)(b+d)(c+d)} \sim \chi^2_1,$$

a Chi-squared distribution with 1 degree of freedom. An approximate one-sided p-value can be calculated using $p - value = P(\chi^2_1 > \chi^2_{ij} | H_0)$. There are suggestions [45] to claim i^{th} AE and j^{th} Drug as a SDR with $\chi^2_{ij} \geq 4, n_{ij} \geq 3$.

Several continuity corrections are made in the calculation of the χ^2 statistic. For example, one may calculate it by using, $\chi^2 = \sum((O - E)^2 - 0.5)/E$, or Yule's $Q = \frac{ad-bc}{ad+bc}$, with cell frequencies a, b, c, d, and that $-1 \leq Q \leq 1$. The 95% CI is given by

$$CI_{Q,100(1-\alpha)\%} = Q \pm z_{1-\alpha/2} \frac{1 - Q^2}{2} \sqrt{\frac{1}{a} + \frac{1}{b} + \frac{1}{c} + \frac{1}{d}}.$$

The Yate's Chi-squared is given by

$$\chi^2_{Yate} = \frac{(|ad - bc| - \frac{1}{2}n^2)n}{(a+b)(a+c)(b+d)(c+d)},$$

where $n = a + b + c + d$.

2.2 Review of Common Bayes and Empirical Bayes Methods

Commonly used Bayesian methods for signal detection from a large database discussed here are: Bayesian Confidence Propagation Neural Network (BCPNN), Multi-item Gamma Poisson Shrinker (MGPS, also known as

Gamma Poissor Shrinker (GPS)), New IC Method, and Simplified Bayes (sB) Method. Some Bayesian methods based on the Logistic and Poisson regression models [55, 105, 106] for analysis of adverse event reports are not discussed here.

2.2.1 Bayesian confidence propagation neural network (BCPNN)

The Bayesian Confidence Propagation Neural Network [22] method for the disproportionality analysis is based on the IC measure because of its derivation from measures used in Information Theory [120], defined as $IC_{ij} = log_2(\frac{p_{ij}}{p_{i.} \times p_{.j}})$. From Table 2.1, for a fixed drug, say $Drug_j$, construct I 2×2 tables, as given above, and assume that

$$\begin{aligned}
&n_{ij}|p_{ij} \sim Bin(n_{..}, p_{ij}) \text{ with } p_{ij} \sim Beta(\alpha_{ij}, \beta_{ij});\\
&n_{i.}|p_{i.} \sim Bin(n_{..}, p_{i.}) \text{ with } p_{i.} \sim Beta(\alpha_{i.}, \beta_{i.});\\
&n_{.j}|p_{.j} \sim Bin(n_{..}, p_{.j}) \text{ with } p_{.j} \sim Beta(\alpha_{.j}, \beta_{.j});
\end{aligned}$$

where $p_{ij}, p_{i.}, p_{.j}$ are independent. Assume further that $\alpha_{ij} = \alpha_{i.} = \beta_{i.} = \alpha_{.j} = \beta_{.j} = 1$ and $\beta_{ij} = \frac{1}{E(p_{i.}|n_{i.})E(p_{.j}|n_{.j})} - 1$. That is, the prior for $p_{i.}$ and $p_{.j}$ are uniform on $(0, 1)$ and that the prior for p_{ij} is an informative and data-dependent prior, $Beta(1, \beta_{ij})$, where β_{ij} is determined by solving the equation that the prior mean of p_{ij} is equal to its posterior mean under the null hypothesis $H_0 : p_{ij} = p_{i.} \times p_{.j}$; β_{ij} is obtained by solving the equation:

$$\frac{1}{1 + \beta_{ij}} = E(p_{i.}|n_{i.})E(p_{.j}|n_{.j}).$$

The posterior distributions of p_{ij}, $p_{i.}$, and $p_{.j}$ are also Beta distributions with updated parameters, namely

$$\begin{aligned}
p_{ij}|n_{ij} &\sim Beta(1 + n_{ij}, 1 + (n_{..} - n_{ij})),\\
p_{i.}|n_{i.} &\sim Beta(1 + n_{i.}, 1 + (n_{..} - n_{i.})),\\
p_{.j}|n_{.j} &\sim Beta(1 + n_{.j}, 1 + (n_{..} - n_{.j})).
\end{aligned}$$

Using these results, $\gamma = \hat{\beta}_{ij} + 1 = \frac{(n_{..}+2)^2}{(n_{i.}+1)(n_{.j}+1)}$. Also, using the delta method,

$$\begin{aligned}
IC_{ij} &= log_2(\frac{p_{ij}}{p_{i.} \times p_{.j}})\\
&\approx \frac{1}{log2}\left\{log\left(\frac{E(p_{ij}|n_{ij})}{E(p_{i.}|n_{i.})E(p_{.j}|n_{.j})}\right) + \frac{(p_{ij} - E(p_{ij}|n_{ij}))}{E(p_{ij}|n_{ij})} - \frac{(p_{i.} - E(p_{i.}|n_{i.}))}{E(p_{i.}|n_{i.})}\right.\\
&\quad \left. - \frac{(p_{.j} - E(p_{.j}|n_{.j}))}{E(p_{.j}|n_{.j})}\right\}
\end{aligned}$$

so that the posterior mean and the variance of IC_{ij} are given by

$$E(IC_{ij}|data) = log_2\left(\frac{E(p_{ij}|n_{ij}, \hat{\beta}_{ij})}{E(p_{i.}|n_{i.})E(p_{.j}|n_{.j})}\right)$$
$$= log_2\frac{(n_{ij}+1)(n_{..}+2)^2}{(n_{..}+\gamma)(n_{i.}+1)(n_{.j}+1)}$$

and

$$Var(IC_{ij}|data) \approx$$
$$\frac{1}{(log2)^2}\left\{\frac{Var(p_{ij}-E(p_{ij}|n_{ij}))}{E(p_{ij}|n_{ij})^2}+\frac{Var(p_{i.}-E(p_{i.}|n_{i.}))}{E(p_{i.}|n_{i.})^2}+\frac{Var(p_{.j}-E(p_{.j}|n_{.j}))}{E(p_{.j}|n_{.j})^2}\right\}$$
$$= \frac{1}{(log_2)^2}\left\{\frac{(n_{..}-n_{ij}+\gamma-1)}{(n_{ij}+1)(n_{..}+\gamma+1)}+\frac{(n_{..}-n_{i.}+1)}{(n_{i.}+1)(n_{..}+3)}+\frac{(n_{..}-n_{.j}+1)}{(n_{.j}+1)(n_{..}+3)}.\right\}$$

Let $IC_{\alpha/2} = E(IC_{ij}|data) - z_{1-\alpha/2}\sqrt{Var(IC_{ij}|data)}$ denote the lower limit of the $100(1-\alpha)\%$ CI for IC_{ij}. Then, the AE_i is a signal for $Drug_j$ if $IC_{\alpha/2} > 0$. Since the hyperparameter β_{ij} is estimated from the data, the BCPNN method is strictly an empirical Bayes method.

Noren et al. [116] extended BCPNN method with IC measures to study higher order associations. Instead of assuming that $n_{ij}, n_{i.}, n_{.j}$ are independent Binomials with probabilities $p_{ij}, p_{i.}, p_{.j}$, respectively, which in turn, are assumed to be independent Beta random variables, the cell counts in a 2×2 table (Table 2.2), (a, b, c, d) are assumed to follow a Multinomial distribution, $Mult((a+b+c+d); p_{11}, p_{10}, p_{01}, p_{00})$, and that the cell probabilities $(p_{11}, p_{10}, p_{01}, p_{00}) \sim Dir(a_{11}, a_{10}, a_{01}, a_{00})$, a Dirichlet distribution. They proposed several modifications and improvements of IC, and presented extensions of IC to third and higher order associations.

2.2.2 Multi-item gamma poisson shrinker (MGPS)

The Multi-item Gamma Poisson Shrinker (MGPS) method or GPS, developed by DuMouchel [41], is based on the assumption that the number of reports n_{ij} for $AE_i, Drug_j), i = 1, \cdots, I; j = 1, \cdots, J$ are independent Poisson random variables with means $\mu_{ij} = \lambda_{ij} \times E_{ij}$, where λ_{ij} denote reporting ratios (i.e., RR_{ij}), and E_{ij} denote expected number of counts under the null hypothesis $H_0 : \lambda_{ij} = 1$. The parameters λ_{ij} are assumed to be independent with a common prior, which is a mixture of two Gamma distributions,

$$\lambda_{ij} \sim P \times Gamma(.|\alpha_1, \beta_1) + (1-P) \times Gamma(.|\alpha_2, \beta_2),$$

where $Gamma(.|\alpha, \beta)$ is a Gamma distribution with mean α/β and variance α/β^2, and $0 \leq P \leq 1$ is the mixing probability. The estimates of the five (unknown) parameters $\alpha_1, \beta_1, \alpha_2, \beta_2, P$ are obtained by their maximum likelihood estimates (MLEs), from the integrated likelihood function. The posterior distributions of λ_{ij} are also a mixture of two Gamma distributions with updated parameters:

$$\lambda_{ij}|data \sim Q\times Gamma(.|\alpha_1+n_{ij}, \beta_1+E_{ij})+(1-Q)\times Gamma(.|\alpha_2+n_{ij}, \beta_2+E_{ij}),$$

with mixing probability Q denoting the posterior probability that the parameter λ_{ij} comes from the first component of the above mixture distribution. This is given by

$$Q = \frac{P \times NB(n_{ij}|\alpha_1, 1/(1+\beta_1/E_{ij}))}{P \times NB(n_{ij}|\alpha_1, 1/(1+\beta_1/E_{ij})) + (1-P) \times NB(n_{ij}|\alpha_2, 1/(1+\beta_2/E_{ij}))},$$

where $NB(x|m,p)$ is a Negative Binomial distribution with parameters m and p. The posterior means and variances of λ_{ij} are as follows:

$$E(\lambda_{ij}|data) = \hat{Q}\frac{\hat{\alpha}_1 + n_{ij}}{\hat{\beta}_1 + E_{ij}} + (1-\hat{Q})\frac{\hat{\alpha}_2 + n_{ij}}{\hat{\beta}_2 + E_{ij}},$$
$$Var(\lambda_{ij}|data) = \hat{Q}\frac{\hat{\alpha}_1 + n_{ij}}{(\hat{\beta}_1 + E_{ij})^2} + (1-\hat{Q})\frac{\hat{\alpha}_2 + n_{ij}}{(\hat{\beta}_2 + E_{ij})^2},$$

where $\hat{Q}, \hat{\alpha}_1, \hat{\alpha}_2, \hat{\beta}_1, \hat{\beta}_2$ are the maximum likelihood estimates. One can also either use the delta method to evaluate $E(log_2\lambda_{ij}|data)$ and $Var(log_2\lambda_{ij}|data)$ or evaluate them directly by integrating with respect to the posterior distribution. Using the delta method,

$$log\lambda_{ij} \approx log\tilde{\lambda} + (\lambda - \tilde{\lambda})\frac{1}{\tilde{\lambda}};$$

hence, taking $\tilde{\lambda} = E(\lambda|data)$,

$$E(log_2(\lambda)|data) \approx log_2 E(\lambda|data);$$

$$Var(log_2(\lambda)|data) \approx \frac{1}{(log2)^2}\frac{Var(\lambda|data)}{(E(\lambda|data))^2};$$

The lower limit of a $100(1-\alpha)\%$ CI of λ_{ij}:

$$EB_{\alpha/2}(\lambda) = \exp\left\{log_2 E(\lambda|data) - z_{1-\alpha/2}\frac{\sqrt{Var(\lambda|data)}}{E(\lambda|data)}\right\}$$
$$= EBGM(\lambda) \times \exp\left\{ - z_{1-\alpha/2}\frac{\sqrt{Var(\lambda|data)}}{E(\lambda|data)}\right\},$$

where $EBGM(\lambda_{ij}) = \exp\{log_2 E(\lambda_{ij}|data)\}$ is the empirical Bayes geometric mean of λ_{ij}. A direct evaluation of $E(log_2(\lambda)|data)$ and $Var(log_2(\lambda)|data)$ can also be carried out as explained in the subsection on the Simplified Bayes Method given below.

The 5th quantile of the sampled λ_{ij} (EB05) from the posterior of λ_{ij} is considered as the measurement score [42], and if EB05 is greater than a threshold value of 2, the pair $AE_i, Drug_j$ is a SDR [133]. A 90% credible intervals for λ_{ij} can also be obtained from (EB05, EB95). The five parameters of the prior are estimated from the whole data, and hence the prior is data-dependent and the method is rightly called an empirical Bayes method. The EBGM can also be used for decision making [20]. Stratified analyses using MGPS method and covariates such as age and gender can also be conducted by calculating expected counts, $E_{ij} = \sum_s E_{ij}^{(s)}$.

As λ_{ij}'s have a common prior, they are assumed a priori exchangeable, an assumption that seems to be quite restrictive, and not easily verifiable. Furthermore, the common prior for λ_{ij}'s leads to the maximum likelihood estimation of the unknown hyperparameters of the two Gamma distributions and the unknown mixing probability by maximizing the integrated likelihood from the entire (large) table.

2.2.3 New IC

The new IC method [116, 114] assumes that the number of reports n_{ij} for $(AE_i, Drug_j), i = 1, \cdots, I, j = 1, \cdots, J$ are independent Poisson random variables with means $\mu_{ij} = \lambda_{ij} \times E_{ij}$, where λ_{ij} denote reporting ratios (i.e., RR_{ij}), and E_{ij} denote expected number of counts under the null hypothesis $H_0 : \lambda_{ij} = 1$, and $log_2\lambda_{ij} = IC_{ij}$.

The parameters λ_{ij} are assumed to be independent with a common prior, $\lambda_{ij} \sim^{iid} Gamma(.|1/2, 1/2)$ with mean 1 and variance 2. The posterior distribution of λ_{ij} is also a Gamma, $\lambda_{ij}|data \sim^{ind} Gamma(.|n_{ij} + 1/2, E_{ij} + 1/2$, so that $E(log_2\lambda_{ij}|data) \approx log_2\frac{n_{ij}+0.5}{E_{ij}+0.5}$. Noren [114] mentioned to obtain the credible interval limits by numerical solutions of

$$\int_0^{\lambda_\alpha} G(d\lambda|n_{ij} + 0.5, E_{ij} + 0.5) = \alpha$$

for $\alpha = 0.025$ and $\alpha = 0.975$. Then, the 95% credible interval for $IC_{new} = log_2\lambda_{ij}$ is $(\lambda_{0.025}, \lambda_{0.975})$. The new IC method can also be used for stratified analysis using $E_{ij} = \sum_s E_{ij}^{(s)}$. In addition, Noren et al. [115] studied drug-drug, and higher order-interactions using $\Omega = log_2\frac{n_{ijk}+0.5}{E_{ijk}+0.5}$.

2.2.4 Simplified Bayes

Simplified Bayesian (sB) method [79] assumes a weaker assumption than the MGPS method on the common prior distribution of λ_{ij}, which are independent and identically distributed with the common prior as $Gamma(c, c)$; i.e., $\lambda_{ij} \sim^{iid} Gamma(c, c)$ with mean 1 and variance $1/c$. Three types of c chosen by Huang et al. [79] were 0.5, 0.01, 0.0001 with a common mean of 1 and variances 2, 100, and 10,000 respectively. The case with $c = 0.5$ can be considered as an informative case, while the other two cases are less informative and non-informative.

In addition, a uniform hyperprior for c ($c \sim U(0, 1)$) can be assigned. This can be considered as a hierarchical simplified Bayesian (HsB) model. The sB method with fixed $c(0 < c < 1)$ is well related to the new IC method [116], which is explained below. The sB method with fixed c is also computationally much less intensive than HsB method and MGPS method. With fixed c, the posterior distribution of λ_{ij} is also Gamma distribution:

$$\lambda_{ij}|n_{ij}, E_{ij} \sim Gamma(c + n_{ij}, c + E_{ij}).$$

Thus, the posterior mean and posterior variance of λ_{ij} are given as: $E(sB_{ij}) = \frac{n_{ij}+c}{E_{ij}+c}$, $Var(sB_{ij}) = \frac{n_{ij}+c}{(E_{ij}+c)^2}$. The lower limit of the 90% CI for λ_{ij} is given by:

$$sB_{c;\alpha=0.05} = \frac{n_{ij}+c}{E_{ij}+c} - 1.645\sqrt{\frac{n_{ij}+c}{(E_{ij}+c)^2}}.$$

One may use the lower limit $sB_{c;\alpha=0.05}$ as the criterion rather than the lower bound of the credible interval of λ_{ij} to be greater than 2 for making the decision for the pair $(AE_i, Drug_j)$ to be a possible SDR.

More details of the relationship between the new IC and sB are included in Appendix 2.4.1.

2.2.5 Poisson-DP method

Bayesian methods assign a common prior distribution to the reporting rates in order to smooth the reporting rates estimated from the data. The common priors, in the available Bayesian or Empirical Bayesian methods, are all specified in a parametric form with unknown hyper-parameters; for example, in the MGPS method [41], the common prior is a mixture of two Gamma distributions with hyper-parameters estimated from the data, and in sB method [79], it is a single Gamma with both the scale and shape parameters specified to be the same and assumed between (0,1). Since the number of signals detected is sensitive to the choice of the priors, irrespective of whether the prior is subjective (pre-specified by the researcher) or objective (estimated from the data), it is preferable to use a nonparametric prior distribution than a parametric one. Poisson-Dirichlet process (DP) method proposed by Hu et al. [74] is a new signal detection methodology based on nonparametric (hierarchical) Bayesian model, in which the common prior, for the reporting rates, is the DP. Characterizations of DP can be found in Refs. [21, 130, 129]. The DP model provides flexibility of modeling the reporting rates of all drug-event combinations without any parametric assumption about the prior distribution.

The parametric priors for λ_{ij}'s, such as a single Gamma distribution in sB method or a mixture of two Gamma distributions in MGPS method, can be relaxed by a non-parametric prior, the DP prior, described as follows:

$$\lambda_{ij}|G \stackrel{iid}{\sim} G,$$

where G is distributed as the $DP(\rho, G_0)$; that is,

$$G|(\rho, G_0) \sim DP(\rho, G_0),$$

with the precision parameter ρ and the baseline distribution G_0. The baseline distribution is, $G_0 = Gamma(\alpha, \alpha)$, a Gamma distribution with mean 1 and variance $1/\alpha$. Further assume that the hyper-priors for the hyper-parameters α and ρ are:

$$\alpha \sim Uniform(0, 1),$$

$$\rho \sim Uniform(0.2, 10),$$

where the lower bound of the ρ is taken to be greater than 0, so that the marginal density of ρ is integrable.

In the above Bayesian hierarchical model, the baseline distribution G_0 is the prior guess of the common unknown distribution, G, of the relative reporting rates λ_{ij}'s, and the precision parameter ρ is the measure of the strength of this belief (probability that G_0 is true G). A large value of ρ indicates that, the prior guess G_0 is very close to G, and that a small value of ρ allows G_0 to deviate more from G. Thus ρ provides a definite information concerning the unknown prior distribution G [130]. Theoretically, it is because a draw from $DP(\rho, G_0)$; that is, from the (random) distribution G, always results a discrete distribution, where the distinct points, in support of G, have the distribution G_0. Small values of ρ cause more repetitions (i.e., ties) of the points in the support of G, and yield less number of distinct points in the support. When ρ converges to 0, G converges to a random degenerate distribution δ_Y where the single support point Y has distribution G_0 [130].

There are two main advantages of assuming the above formulation of λ_{ij}'s. First, the modeling of λ_{ij}'s using the DP prior leads to more flexibility in the underlying distribution G to be the nonparametric. That is, compared to the sB and HsB methods with a single Gamma prior, and the MGPS method with a mixture of two Gamma priors, the DP prior allows the availability of a much richer class of distributions, thereby better accommodating lack of knowledge of the distributional structure of the relative reporting rates, λ_{ij}'s. Second, the draws from G are discrete values, resulting in possible ties (clusters). In the FAERS database, we believe that the drugs from the same class share some common adverse events. Thus, the natural clustering property of the DP is helpful in ascertaining clusters of drug-event combinations that have the same relative reporting rate.

Furthermore, it is reasonable to assume that different drugs or drug classes share different prior information, i.e., different precision parameters and baseline distributions, which brings more flexibility to the DP model. Thus, for a specific j^{th} Drug, the DP prior can be described as follows:

$$\lambda_{ij} | G_j \overset{iid}{\sim} G_j,$$

where G_j is distributed as the $DP(\rho_j, G_{0j})$; that is,

$$G_j | (\rho_j, G_{0j}) \sim DP(\rho_j, G_{0j}),$$

with the precision parameter ρ_j and the baseline distribution G_{0j}. The baseline distribution is, $G_{0j} = Gamma(\alpha_j, \alpha_j)$, and the hyper- priors for the hyper-parameters α_j and ρ_j are:

$$\alpha_j \sim Uniform(0, 1),$$

$$\rho_j \sim Uniform(0.2, 10).$$

Computationally, this formulation allows the detection of adverse events (AE signals) by drug.

There are two ways to implement the DP prior: Polya-urn representation of the DP [24], and constructive definition of DP [130, 129]. The details of the Polya-urn representation of the DP are described in Appendix 2.4.2.

The constructive definition of the DP is well known as stick-breaking definition. The MCMC algorithms are as follows:

$$G_j(.) = \sum_{l=1}^{\infty} w_l \delta_{\theta_l},$$

$$\theta_l \overset{iid}{\sim} G_{0j}(.),$$

$$w_1 = v_1, w_r = v_r \prod_{s=1}^{r-1}(1 - v_s), r \geq 2, \quad \text{and} \quad v_s \overset{iid}{\sim} Beta(1, \rho_j), s \geq 1,$$

where δ_θ denotes the degenerate distribution with all its mass at θ. In practice, we can truncate the above mixture at some finite number L with $w_L = 1 - \sum_{l=1}^{L-1} w_l$, where L is usually taken to be the square root of the sample size or the logarithm of the sample size. Hence, $G \approx \sum_{l=1}^{L} w_l \delta_{\theta_l}$ after the truncation. The advantage of this finite truncation mixture representation of the DP model is that, the MCMC samples can be generated using the standard MCMC procedures. A drug-event combination (i, j) is detected as a signal of disproportionate reporting (SDR), if the 5th quartile of the sampled λ_{ij} is greater than a threshold value of 2. This threshold is the same as that in the MGPS method.

From the simulation study comparing the Frequentist and Bayesian methods included in Ref. [74], LRT method (detailed in Chapter 3) has been proven to control FDR and is superior to the Poisson-DP method because this DP method tends to be more conservative. The advantage of the Poisson-DP method is that the nonparametric nature of the DP model helps with the clustering of AEs within each drug as the samples from a DP are discrete with probability one, and distinct values represent different clusters of AEs.

2.3 Notes and Discussion

- Use of the Frequentist and Bayesian methods

The Frequentist and Bayesian statistical methods (with unified notations), for signal detection using large safety data are presented in this chapter. Many of these methods use 2×2 contingency tables formed by a particular drug vs. rest of the drugs crossed with a particular AE vs. rest of the AEs. Some drugs in the " rest of the drugs" column (or some AEs in the "rest of the AEs" row) may be correlated with the particular drug (or AE). The methods discussed here do not account for this correlation. Therefore, these signal detection methods are usually used for hypothesis generation.

- Note on the Bayesian methods

  The MGPS method works on a large data-matrix, the entire $I \times J$ table, and uses a common mixture prior. Unlike the BCPNN method, which is also an empirical Bayes method, and involves the estimation of one parameter associated with each 2×2 table, the estimation of the parameters, from the integrated likelihood based on the entire data, is computationally intensive. New IC, sB, HsB, and Poisson-DP methods are fully Bayesian methods, with informative or non-informative priors, and are easy to compute with pre-specified priors and their closed forms of the posterior distributions. Because of borrowing information from the entire data, such empirical and fully Bayesian methods result in the Bayes estimates of the relative reporting ratios of each drug-AE pair, that have shrinkage to the null hypothesis (no association between drugs and AEs). However, these methods also produce false positive signals; although their extent is not clear and varies with different data.

- Regression models

  Most of the methods discussed in this chapter work on aggregated data generated from individual-level data. To evaluate the effect of variables such as drug class, stratification, and interactions, it is more appropriate to consider regression models. However, the computational complexity is very intensive, and sometimes the complete data are not available. The type-I error and FDR may not be controlled for these regression methods for comparing multiple drugs and AEs.

- Note on stratified analysis

  Stratified analysis approaches have been discussed for some Frequentist and Bayesian methods. These include LRT, sB, new IC, HsB, Poisson-DP, and MGPS. Other methods, such as PRR and ROR can also account for strata using Mantel-Haenszel method [73], producing corresponding p-values and confidence intervals. The presence or absence of signals may be affected by stratification. Woo et al. [140] compared stratified PRR and EB05 (the lower bound of 90% CI)) measures and discussed the importance of strata for computation of appropriate disproportionality statistics. Note that some confounding factors with less missing values (such as gender, and age) can be adjusted by stratified analyses. However, not many drug safety databases (collected through spontaneous reporting system) include sufficient information for stratified analyses on confounders.

- Literature for methods comparison

  Comparisons of some of the data mining methods have been done in the literature. For example, Roux et al. [125] compared several Frequentist and Bayesian methods for data mining using simulation, but with limited number of drugs and AEs. Banks et al [20] studied MGPS (two measures: EBGM (the geometric mean) and EB05 (the lower bound of 90% CI)) and PRR in the VARES database. Ahmed et al. [16] used two simulation procedures to compare the false-positive performances for the reporting odds ratio (ROR), the information component (IC), the gamma Poisson shrinkage (GPS), and also for two FDR-based methods derived from the GPS model and Fisher's test. Huang et al. [77] reviewed commonly used statistical methods in surveillance and described the relationship among the methods with unified notations. Ding et al. [38] reviewed several statistical methods for signal detection that are mostly in use in post-marketing safety surveillance of spontaneously reported AEs via intensive simulation and made recommendations.

- Decision criteria and FDR-based methods

  Most of the known methods discussed in this chapter are not designed for analyzing multiple AEs for signals simultaneously. The null hypothesis is that there is no association between a drug and an AE. If the hypothesis is about only one drug-AE combination, the type-I error is well-controlled at a given α level. However, in cases with many drug-AE combinations of interest, these methods do not control the overall type-I error in the presence of multiple comparisons and result in too many false-positive alarms.

  All these methods (except the regression-based methods) are based on a 2×2 contingency table wherein a particular drug-AE combination is considered. These methods generate a score for each drug-AE combination and compare the scores with a threshold. A score exceeding the threshold indicates a strong association between the specific drug and AE. For example, the decision rule for determination of a SDR is usually based on the lower limit of the 95% CI of the parameters exceeding a pre-specified threshold value (such as 1.0 for PRR or ROR, and 0 for IC). However, these thresholds may not be of clinical importance in which case a higher value of thresholds such as 1.2 (20% increase of reporting rate) or 2 (twice the reporting rate) may be more relevant for PRR [133]. Moreover, increasing the threshold value may reduce the number of false-positive alarms [69, 70]. Hauben et al. 2007 [70] also suggests that additional criterion based on cell counts (such as n_{ij} greater than 2) may reduce the number of signals detected, and in turn may reduce the FDR.

These thresholds commonly used are a trade-off between generating too many "false positive signals" if the threshold value is too small, and missing "true positive signals" if it is too large. The specification of the threshold is subjective [35] and the effect of varying thresholds on the type-I error and false discovery rate (FDR) has not been systematically studied and reported in the literature.

Another approach for overall type-I error control is to use Bonferroni correction formula for preserving the overall type-I error; however, with the number of AEs in large post-market safety databases being large, the Bonferroni correction (https://en.wikipedia.org/wiki/Bonferroni_correction) would be very conservative. Benjamini-Hochberg (B-H) procedure [23] may also be used to control the type-I error, which is often used in genomics applications. Ahmed et al. [17, 16] described the use of B-H procedure in pharmacovigilance applications. In addition, they developed a decision rule that is based on FDR to offset the false discovery problem. Ding et al. [38] summarized and evaluated the FDR-based methods and mentioned that the FDR criterion-based methods, FDR-PRR and FDR-ROR offer very little improvement in otherwise unacceptably high FDR; only FDR-BCPNN controls FDR fairly well at the cost of lower power and sensitivity.

- Methods for active surveillance

  The statistical methods, including the modifications of the data mining methods, for signal detection in longitudinal observational databases (called active surveillance) are not discussed in detail in this chapter. Some developments and literature are summarized below.

  The Observational Medical Outcomes Partnership (OMOP), a public and private partnership chaired by the FDA, and managed through the NIH, conducts methodological research on active drug safety surveillance to inform the national drug safety efforts by evaluating the performance of methods across a network of 10 databases covering over 200 million patient lives [106]. OMOP has built a library of methods that can be found at https://fnih.org/what-we-do/major-completed-programs/omop, and include disproportionality analysis methods and methods for active surveillance.

  In May 2008, FDA launched the Sentinel Initiative to develop and implement an electronic safety system called the Sentinel System. This system was established for monitoring the safety of FDA-regulated medical products by leveraging existing electronic healthcare data in partnership with organizations such as academic medical centers, healthcare systems, and health insurance companies. The Sentinel System is focused on developing active safety surveillance for FDA-approved medical products (e.g., drugs, biologics, and devices) which involves signal detection or generation, refinement, and validation. The special issue of Pharmacoepidemiology and

Drug Safety, Volume 21 [121] is fully devoted to the articles on the FDA Sentinel System, and includes sequential methods for active safety surveillance by Cook et al. [32].

Additionally, Noren et al. [114] (29) applied the New IC method (discussed in Section 2.2.3) to study the temporal pattern discovery in longitudinal electronic patient records. Schumie [128] proposed a Longitudinal Gamma Poisson Shrinker (LGPS) method for signal detection from OMOP longitudinal observational data with exposure-time information. Kulldorff et al. [96] developed the maximum sequential probability ratio test (maxSPRT) method for active surveillance for vaccine safety data. Li [102] proposed a conditional sequential sampling procedure for drug safety surveillance. Longitudinal LRT methods [81] for active surveillance are also presented in Chapter 6. For details on other methods for longitudinal safety databases, see Ref. [150].

2.4 Appendix

2.4.1 Relationship between new IC and sB methods

The sB has a simple relation with New IC that is given by (using the delta method):

$$E(IC_{New}) \approx log_2 \frac{n_{ij}+0.5}{E_{ij}+0.5} = log_2(sB_{0.5});$$

$$Var(IC_{New}|data) \approx \frac{1}{(log2)^2}\frac{Var(sB_{0.5})}{(E(sB_{0.5}))^2}$$

$$= \frac{1}{(log2)^2}\frac{1}{(n_{ij}+0.5)},$$

so that the lower limit of the 95% CI for IC_{New} is:

$$log_2 \frac{n_{ij}+0.5}{E_{ij}+0.5} - 1.96\frac{1}{log2}\sqrt{\frac{1}{n_{ij}+0.5}}.$$

The exact evaluation of $E(IC_{New}|data)$ and $Var(IC_{New}|data)$ can be carried out directly as follows:

$$E(IC_{New}|data) = \frac{1}{log2}\int (log\lambda)G^*(d\lambda),$$

where $G^*(.) = Gamma(.|n^*, E^*)$, with $n^* = n + 0.5, E^* = E + 0.5$. Define

$\lambda^* = \lambda \times E^*$. Then

$$\int (log\lambda)G^*(d\lambda) = \frac{1}{\Gamma(n^*)}\int (log\lambda^*)G^*(d\lambda^*) - log(E^*)$$
$$= \frac{d(log\Gamma(n^*))}{dn^*} - log(E^*) = \psi(n^*) - log(E^*),$$

so that $E(IC_{New}|data) = \frac{1}{log2}(\psi(n^*) - log(E^*)$, where $\psi(n^*)$ is a digamma function. Similarly,

$$\int (log\lambda)^2 G^*(d\lambda) = \frac{1}{\Gamma(n^*)}\int (log\lambda^*)^2 G^*(d\lambda^*) + (log(E^*))^2 - 2(log(E^*)\psi(n^*)$$
$$= \frac{\Gamma''(n^*)}{\Gamma(n^*)} + (log(E^*))^2 - 2(log(E^*))\psi(n^*);$$

so that

$$Var(IC_{New}|data) = \frac{1}{(log2)^2}\left\{\frac{\Gamma''(n^*)}{\Gamma(n^*)} + (log(E^*))^2 - 2(log(E^*))\psi(n^*) - (\psi(n^*) - log(E^*))^2\right\}$$
$$= \frac{1}{(log2)^2}\left\{\frac{\Gamma''(n^*)}{\Gamma(n^*)} - \psi^2(n^*)\right\}$$
$$= \frac{1}{(log2)^2}\frac{d^2(log\Gamma(n^*))}{dn^{*2}} = \frac{1}{(log2)^2}\psi_1(n^*),$$

where $psi_1(n^*)$ is the trigamma function.

2.4.2 Polya-urn representation of the Dirichlet process prior—Conditional distributions

For Polya urn Representation of the Dirichlet Process (DP) prior, the joint distribution of the λ_{ij}'s, conditional on G_{0j}'s and ρ_j's, is given by

$$\pi(\lambda_{11}, \lambda_{12}, ..., \lambda_{1J}, \lambda_{21}, ..., \lambda_{IJ}) =$$
$$\prod_{i=1}^{I}\prod_{j=1}^{J}\left[\frac{\rho_j}{\rho_j + l_{ij}}G(d\lambda_{ij}) + \frac{1}{\rho_j + l_{ij} - 1}\sum_{l_{i'j'} < l_{ij}} \delta_{\lambda_{i'j'}}(d\lambda_{ij})\right].$$

Here, we sort the list of $\{\lambda_{ij}, i = 1, ..., I, j = 1, ..., J\}$ as $\{\lambda_{11}, \lambda_{12}, ..., \lambda_{1J}, \lambda_{21}, ..., \lambda_{IJ}\}$. l_{ij} represents the order number of λ_{ij} in the list of λ's, and $l_{i'j'} < l_{ij}$ means $\lambda_{i'j'}$ is before λ_{ij}. Because of the exchangeability of the λ_{ij}'s, we can write the conditional distributions of any λ_{ij} given the rest of other λ's, ρ_j, and α_j as

$$\lambda_{ij}|\{\lambda_{i'j'}, i' \neq i \quad \text{or} \quad j' \neq j, \alpha_j, \rho_j\}$$
$$\sim \frac{\rho_j}{\rho_j + IJ - 1}G(d\lambda_{ij}) + \frac{1}{\rho_j + IJ - 1}\sum_{l=1}^{L_{ij}} \delta_{\lambda^*_{ijl}(d\lambda_{ij})},$$

where $\{\lambda^*_{ijl}, l = 1, ..., L_{ij}\}$ are the distinct atoms of $\{\lambda_{i'j'}, (i', j') \neq (i, j)\}$ and $\{p_{ijl}\}$ are the multiplicities of λ^*_{ijl}. Let $\boldsymbol{\theta} = (\lambda_{ij}, i = 1, ..., L_{ij}, j = 1, ..., J, \alpha_j, \rho_j)$. Then, the likelihood function and the posterior distribution of $\boldsymbol{\theta}$ are as follows:

$$\begin{aligned} L(data|\boldsymbol{\theta}) &= \prod_{i=1}^{I}\prod_{j=1}^{J} p(n_{ij}|\boldsymbol{\theta}) \\ &\propto \prod_{i=1}^{I}\prod_{j=1}^{J} \frac{exp(-\lambda_{ij}E_{ij})(\lambda_{ij}E_{ij})^{n_{ij}}}{n_{ij}!}, \end{aligned}$$

$$\begin{aligned} \pi_{post}(\boldsymbol{\theta}|data) &= L(data|\boldsymbol{\theta})\pi(\boldsymbol{\theta}) \\ &= \prod_{i=1}^{I}\prod_{j=1}^{J} p(n_{ij}|\boldsymbol{\theta})\pi(\lambda_{ij}, i{=}1, ..., I, j{=}1, ..., J|\alpha_j, \rho_j)\pi(\alpha_j)\pi(\rho_j). \end{aligned}$$

Furthermore, the (full) conditional distributions of all the parameters are as derived below.

A Markov chain Monte Carlo (MCMC) procedure, such as the Gibbs sampling, can be implemented, on these conditionals to draw samples from the posterior distribution of $\boldsymbol{\theta}$. However, since the conditional distributions are not analytically tractable, it is still difficult to use this method in computation.

$$\begin{aligned} &\pi(\lambda_{ij}|rest) \\ &\propto p(n_{ij}|\lambda_{ij}, \alpha_j, \rho_j)\pi(\lambda_{i'j'}, (i', j') \neq (i, j), \alpha_j, \rho_j) \\ &\propto \frac{exp(-\lambda_{ij}E_{ij})(\lambda_{ij}E_{ij})^{n_{ij}}}{n_{ij}!}\Big(\frac{\rho_j}{\rho_j + IJ - 1}g(\lambda_{ij}|\alpha_j, \alpha_j) + \frac{1}{\rho_j + IJ - 1}\sum_{l=1}^{L_{ij}} p_{ijl}\delta_{\lambda^*_{ijl}}(d\lambda_{ij})\Big) \\ &\propto \frac{\rho_j}{\rho_j + IJ - 1}E_{ij}^{\alpha_j}\binom{n_{ij} + \alpha_j - 1}{\alpha_j}\Big(\frac{\alpha_j}{\alpha_j + E_{ij}}\Big)^{\alpha_j}\Big(\frac{E_{ij}}{\alpha_j + n_{ij}}\Big)^{n_{ij}} g(\lambda_{ij}|\alpha_j + n_{ij}, \alpha_j + E_{ij}) \\ &+ \frac{1}{\rho_j + IJ - 1}\sum_{l=1}^{L_{ij}} p_{ijl}\frac{exp(-\lambda^*_{ijl}E_{ij})(\lambda^*_{ijl}E_{ij})^{n_{ij}}}{n_{ij}!} \end{aligned}$$

$$\pi(\alpha_j|rest) = \prod_{i=1}^{I}\left(\frac{\rho_j}{\rho_j + IJ - 1}g(\lambda_{ij}|\alpha_j, \alpha_j) + \frac{1}{\rho_j + IJ - 1}\sum_{l=1}^{L_{ij}} p_{ijl}\delta_{\lambda^*_{ijl}(d\lambda_{ij})}\right)\delta_{(0,1)}(\alpha_j)$$

$$\pi(\rho_j|rest) = \prod_{i=1}^{I}\left(\frac{\rho_j}{\rho_j + IJ - 1}g(\lambda_{ij}|\alpha_j, \alpha_j) + \frac{1}{\rho_j + IJ - 1}\sum_{l=1}^{L_{ij}} p_{ijl}\delta_{\lambda^*_{ijl}(d\lambda_{ij})}\right)\delta_{(0.2,10)}(\rho_j),$$

where $g(\lambda_{ij}|\alpha_j, \alpha_j) = \frac{\alpha_j^{\alpha_j}}{\Gamma(\alpha_j)}exp(-\lambda_{ij}\alpha_j)\lambda_{ij}^{\alpha_j - 1}$.

3

Basic LRT Method

When mining in the FAERS data for signals, reviewers, and researchers are usually interested in the following two issues: (1) Identifying the AEs with high reporting rates compared to other AEs associated with a particular drug (Issue 1), and (2) Identifying drugs associated with high reporting rate of a particular AE compared to the other drugs (Issue 2). Huang et al. [80] proposed a likelihood ratio test (LRT) approach for testing the hypothesis for Issue 1 or for Issue 2. LRT has been widely used in cancer surveillance for detecting clusters of high incidence/mortality, [78, 94, 137]. In the basic LRT method, the counts in the drug-event combinations are modeled as Poisson random variables. The threshold for the LRT statistic is determined using a Monte Carlo (MC) simulation procedure, and the test statistic is shown to control both the type-I error and false discovery rates. For illustration, this method is applied to two real data sets obtained from FAERS. Covariate adjustment is described in the analysis to account for possible confounding factors such as age, gender, and race.

3.1 Method Development

In practice, medical officers usually investigate drugs or medical products in the context of Issue 1, because the patient populations are more homogeneous. When comparing several drugs for one AE (Issue 2), one has to exercise caution in terms of clinical interpretation because some drugs may not have a biologically plausible relationship with a particular AE and the patient population may be very heterogeneous especially regarding disease conditions and comorbidities. However, it is useful to compare drugs and products in the same drug class or for the similar indication from the perspectives of class labeling and comparative safety and effectiveness. If one product has higher reporting rate for a critical AE (e.g., liver failure) compared with other products in the same drug class, investigators will explore the reason and consider providing warning message to the public, if necessary. In this case, Issue 2 becomes the focus of interest of the investigators.

In the following sections, the first issue is described in detail, the related test statistic is developed, and is modified to address the second issue. In most of the spontaneous reporting safety databases, there is no valid exposure information or information for the total number of subjects taking a particular drug. Therefore, the methods discussed in this chapter are all developed for investigating the relative reporting rate instead of relative risk. LRT methods incorporating exposure information for relative risk evaluation for safety signal detection using datasets emerging from clinical trials and FAERS are discussed in Chapter 6.

3.1.1 Derivation of likelihood ratio test statistic

Let "AE" be the row variable, and "drug" be the column variable. There are a total of I AEs and J drugs. The cell count n_{ij} is the number of cases reported for the ith AE and j^{th} Drug combination during a selected time period. The total number of reported cases for i^{th} AE is $n_{i.}$ (marginal total for i^{th} row), and the total number of reported cases for j^{th} Drug is $n_{.j}$ (the marginal total for j^{th} column), with $n_{..}$ as the grand total.

The $I \times J$ table (Table 2.1) can be collapsed into multiple 2×2 tables. For a fixed drug $(j*)$, there are I tables, each associated with an AE $(i = 1, ..., I)$. We assume that $n_{ij*} \sim Poisson(n_{i.} \times p_i)$, where p_i is the reporting rate of j*th drug for i^{th} AE; and $(n_{.j*} - n_{ij*}) \sim Poisson((n_{..} - n_{i.}) \times q_i)$, where q_i is the reporting rate of j*th drug for other AEs combined excluding i^{th} AE. Here, the notational dependence of p_i and q_i on j*th drug has been suppressed. In order to investigate the first issue, the null hypothesis (H_0) is defined, as $p_i = q_i = p_0$ (or $rr_i = \frac{p_i}{q_i} = 1$) for all i. The rr can be considered as relative reporting rate here.

Under the null hypothesis, the maximum likelihood estimates for p_0 is $\hat{p}_0 = \frac{n_{.j*}}{n_{..}}$, and the expected number of cases for i^{th} AE and j*th drug is $E_{ij*} = n_{i.} \times \frac{n_{.j*}}{n_{..}} = \frac{n_{i.} n_{.j*}}{n_{..}}$.

Under the two-sided alternative hypothesis ($p_i \neq q_i$ or $rr_i \neq 1$ for at least one i), the maximum likelihood estimates (MLEs) for p_i and q_i (maximized over the unrestricted space of p_i and q_i) are $\hat{p}_i = \frac{n_{ij*}}{n_{i.}}$, and $\hat{q}_i = \frac{n_{.j*} - n_{ij*}}{n_{..} - n_{i.}}$, respectively.

The maximum likelihoods under both the null and the two-sided alternative hypotheses associated with Issue 1 are obtained by replacing the parameters with their MLEs in the likelihood functions, leading to the likelihood ratio, for i^{th} AE and fixed j*th drug,

$$LR_{ij*} = \frac{L_a(\hat{p}_i, \hat{q}_i)}{L_0(\hat{p}_0)} = \frac{\left(\frac{n_{ij*}}{n_{i.}}\right)^{n_{ij*}} \left(\frac{n_{.j*} - n_{ij*}}{n_{..} - n_{i.}}\right)^{(n_{.j*} - n_{ij*})}}{\left(\frac{n_{.j*}}{n_{..}}\right)^{n_{.j*}}}, i = 1, \cdots, I. \tag{3.1}$$

The likelihood ratio test statistic for testing $H_0 : p_i = q_i$ for all AEs, versus, $H_a : p_i \neq q_i$ for at least one AE, is the maximum likelihood ratio

$$MLR = max_i(LR_{ij*}) = max_i \frac{\left(\frac{n_{ij*}}{n_{i.}}\right)^{n_{ij*}} \left(\frac{n_{.j*} - n_{ij*}}{n_{..} - n_{i.}}\right)^{(n_{.j*} - n_{ij*})}}{\left(\frac{n_{.j*}}{n_{..}}\right)^{n_{.j*}}},$$

where the maximum is over AEs $i = 1, ..., I$. For computational convenience, one can work with the log likelihood ratio (LLR), $log(LR_{ij*})$, a monotone function of LR_{ij*}, such that the test statistic MLLR is $max_i[log(LR_{ij*})]$.

For the one-sided alternative hypothesis $p_i > q_i$ (or $rr_i > 1$), the function (3.1) is multiplied by $I(\hat{p_i} > \hat{q_i})$, which is usually the focus of safety signal detection. In this case, the AEs detected as signals have higher reporting rate of jth Drug compared with other AEs.

Note that to address the second issue, one can let AE be the column variable and drug be the row variable, in the above derivation.

3.1.2 MLR incorporating covariate information

The above maximum likelihood ratio (MLR) test statistic uses the information about the drugs, AEs, and the associated counts, but not about any covariates. However, the detected safety signal may be related to factors such as gender and age. For example, a signal for death associated with a particular drug may result from higher reporting rates in males compared to females. Therefore, the MLR test statistic can be constructed by incorporating information on covariates such as gender and age.

Reparametrizing the likelihood ratio LR_{ij*} in (3.1) as function of the expected number of cases E_{ij*} for the ith AE and j*th drug, under the null hypothesis, we obtain

$$LR_{ij} = (\frac{n_{ij*}}{E_{ij*}})^{n_{ij*}}(\frac{n_{.j*} - n_{ij*}}{n_{.j*} - E_{ij*}})^{(n_{.j*} - n_{ij*})} \tag{3.2}$$

$$MLR = max_i LR_{ij} = max_i\big[(\frac{n_{ij*}}{E_{ij*}})^{n_{ij*}}(\frac{n_{.j*} - n_{ij*}}{n_{.j*} - E_{ij*}})^{(n_{.j*} - n_{ij*})}\big], \tag{3.3}$$

and $MLLR = max_i log(LR_{ij})$.

The expected number of cases for i^{th} AE and j*th drug, adjusted for the covariate effect, is

$$E_{ij*} = \sum_m E^m_{ij*} = \sum_m [n^m_{i.} \times \frac{n^m_{.j*}}{n^m_{..}}], \tag{3.4}$$

where m is the number of groups determined by the covariates.

This approach can be extended to adjust for multiple covariates. However, one must note that larger the number of covariates and strata, lesser will be the observed number of cases for each stratum. Another approach for covariate adjustment is to obtain weighted average of LogLR values from different strata based on the covariates. Further details are discussed in Section 5.4.

3.1.3 Hypothesis testing

The distribution of MLLR under H_0, is not analytically tractable, and is obtained using Monte Carlo simulation. First, the number of cases for each AE, for a given j*th drug, are simulated under H_0. Under H_0, since $n_{1j*}, \cdots, n_{Ij*}$ given the margin totals $n_{1.}, \cdots, n_{I.}$, are independent, $Poisson(n_{i.}p_0), i = 1, ..., I$, the joint distribution of $(n_{1j*}, \cdots, n_{Ij*})$, conditioning on $n_{.j*}$ and $(n_{1.}, \cdots, n_{I.})$ is

$$(n_{1j*}, \cdots, n_{Ij*})|n_{.j*}; n_{1.}, \cdots, n_{I.} \sim Multinomial(n_{.j*}, (\eta_1 \frac{n_{1.}}{n_{..}}, \cdots, \eta_I \frac{n_{I.}}{n_{..}})), \tag{3.5}$$

where $\eta_i = 1, i = 1, \cdots, I$. The datasets generated from the above equation have relative reporting rate (rr) for row $i*$ as the following:

$$rr_{i*} = \frac{\eta_{i*} \times \frac{n_{i*.}}{n_{..}} \times n_{.j*}/n_{i*.}}{\sum_{i \neq i*}(\eta_i \times \frac{n_{i.}}{n_{..}} \times n_{.j*})/(n_{..} - n_{i*.})} = \frac{\eta_{i*} \times n_{i*.}}{\sum_{i \neq i*} \eta_i n_{i.}} \frac{\sum_{i \neq i*} n_i}{n_{i*.}} = 1, \tag{3.6}$$

where $\eta_i = 1, i = 1, \cdots, I$.

A total of 9,999 datasets under H_0 are simulated from the Multinomial distribution, and 10,000 MLLRs are calculated (9,999 from the simulated datasets and one from the observed dataset). The null hypothesis is rejected at the $\alpha = 0.05$ level if the value of MLLR from the observed dataset is greater than the 95th percentile of the 10,000 MlLR values (objective threshold). The corresponding p-value is then $pvalue = 1 - R/(1 + 9999)$, where R is the rank of the MLLR value for the observed dataset among all the 10,000 MLLR values. Equivalently, one can also calculate p-value as $pvalue = \frac{\#\text{MLLR from simulation} \geq \text{MLLR from the observed data}}{10{,}000}$.

If the p-value of the MLLR for the observed dataset is less than 0.05 (a pre-specified level of significance), then the drug associated with the MLLR has the (strongest) signal for the j*th AE under consideration. The Monte Carlo-based p-value is exact such that the probability of observing a p-value less than or equal to p is exactly p under the null hypothesis [43]. Having found the AE with the MLLR as a signal, one can also find the AEs that provide the second largest likelihood ratio, the third largest likelihood ratio, etc., and declare them as signals using a step down process as described below.

The likelihood ratio test statistic values $log(LR_{ij*})$ for the observed dataset can be ranked from the largest to the smallest (ordered from 1 to I). After the AE associated with the largest value of the likelihood ratio test statistic (MLLR) is identified as a signal (p-value < 0.05), and H_0 is rejected, one can move to the AE with the second largest value of the likelihood ratio test statistic (i.e., ranked 2nd), determine its p-value from the empirical null distribution of MLLR values obtained using Monte Carlo simulation, and if this p-value is smaller than 0.05, declare the corresponding AE as a signal and move to the next AE associated with the third largest value of the likelihood ratio test statistic, and so on. The likelihood ratio test statistic values from the observed dataset are always compared with the MLLR values from the empirical null distribution for p-value determination. This method with the step-down process controls the overall family wise type-I error at (α) level.

For all methods of investigating safety signals, including the proposed LRT method, the false discovery rate (FDR) is one of the most important measures of performance. FDR is defined by

$$E(\frac{V}{V+S}) = E(\frac{V}{R}),$$

where V is the number of false positives (signals detected incorrectly), S is the number of true positives (signals detected correctly), and R is the total number of signals detected. $\frac{V}{R}$ is defined to be 0, when $R = 0$. The minimum value for FDR is 0 when $V = 0$ (i.e., when no signal is detected incorrectly). Under H_0, $\frac{V}{R} = 1$ for any values of $V > 0$. Then

$$E(\frac{V}{R}|H_0) = 1 \times P(\text{reject } H_0|H_0) = \alpha.$$

Also under H_a, $\frac{V}{R} \leq 1$, if any signals are detected, $E(\frac{V}{R}|H_a) \leq E(\frac{V}{R}|H_0) = \alpha$. Therefore, FDR is always less than or equal to α for LRT method.

3.2 Simulation

In this section, we compare PRR, BCPNN (discussed in Chapter 2), and LRT methods using the performance characteristics: power, type-I error rate, sensitivity, and FDR.

In a simulation study conducted by Ahmed et al. [17], MGPS and BCPNN methods show close performance. However, the derived operating characteristics cannot be generalized since they are specific to a database. This is compounded by the fact that a simulation study for MGPS method requires generation of the entire $I \times J$ matrix for the estimation of the prior parameters and the number of signals detected. In addition, the gamma mixture prior distribution may not be appropriate for every dataset (manifested as non-convergence of the associated algorithm) according to Ding et al. [38]. The multiple parameters associated with this prior distribution provide more variability that may be appropriate for some datasets but not for others. Due to the complex data generation and convergence issue, MGPS method is not included in the simulation study.

3.2.1 Data simulation

Multiple datasets are simulated to reflect the marginal counts from two real-data examples (additional details of the data are discussed in Section 3.3). The first example of the drug Montelukast with 24 AEs represents a dataset with a small number of drug-event combinations, and the second example of the drug Heparin with 1401 AEs represents a dataset with large number of drug-event combinations. The purpose of the examples is to identify possible AE signals (among the AEs with reports) with high relative reporting rate for a single drug (Montelukast or Heparin). Since the study of interest is related to Issue 1, the row variable is AE and the column variable is drug in the simulation study and in the applications. Under the null hypothesis, the data are simulated using (3.5), and under the alternative hypothesis (the rr values not homogeneous with common value equal to 1), the data are simulated using the following:

$$\begin{aligned}&(n_{1j*},\cdots,n_{Ij*})|n_{.j*};n_{1.},\cdots,n_{I.}\\&\sim Multinomial(n_{.j*},(\eta_1\times r_0\times\frac{n_{1.}}{n_{..}},\cdots,\eta_I\times r_0\times\frac{n_{I.}}{n_{..}})),\end{aligned}\tag{3.7}$$

with the constraint that $0\leq\eta_i\times r_0\times\frac{n_{i.}}{n_{..}}\leq 1$, and $\sum_{i=1}^{I}\eta_i\times r_0\times\frac{n_{i.}}{n_{..}}=1$; $j*$ indicates the fixed column for study (the column of Montelukast or the column of Heparin). Here, r_0 can be interpreted as the baseline rate, which may vary with different datasets. The relative reporting rate for row $i*$ is

$$rr_{i*}=\frac{\eta_{i*}\times n_{i*.}}{\sum_{i\neq i*}\eta_i n_{i.}}\frac{\sum_{i\neq i*}n_{i.}}{n_{i*.}}=\eta_{i*},\tag{3.8}$$

where $\eta_i=1$ for all $i\neq i*$. If there are some $\eta_i>1$ for some $i\neq i*$ and $\eta_{i*}=1$, then $rr_{i*}<\eta_{i*}(=1)$.

In the simulations, the values of η are defined as follows: the selected AEs are designated as true signals and are assigned values of η higher than 1 and other not selected AEs are assigned values of η equal to 1. In the data with single true signal (row $i*$), $rr_{i*}=\eta_{i*}>1$, and $rr_i=1, i\neq i*$.

Note that one way of simulating the data without estimating r_0 is to define $r_0=\frac{n_{..}}{\sum_{i=1}^{I}\eta_i n_{i.}}$.

Then the data can be simulated using the following formula:

$$(n_{1j*},\cdots,n_{Ij*})|n_{.j*}\sim Mult(n_{.j*},(\eta_1\frac{n_{1.}}{\sum_{i=1}^{I}(\eta_i n_{i.})},\cdots,\eta_I\frac{n_{I.}}{\sum_{i=1}^{I}(\eta_i n_{i.})})),\tag{3.9}$$

where $\sum_{i=1}^{I}[\eta_i\frac{n_{i.}}{\sum_i^I(\eta_i n_{i.})}]=1$.

The simulation is carried out to study how the η values, the sample size, and the number of signals affect the performance of the methods under comparison by varying the simulation parameters as follows: first, the datasets are simulated with just one AE as a signal and with different corresponding marginal total values for the selected AE signal (small values such as 327 in the first example and 570 in the second example, or moderately large values such as 2108 in the first example and 2103 in the second example). Next, the simulation is carried out to evaluate the case where multiple AEs are signals with homogeneous(same) $\eta(>1)$ values by simulating datasets with 5 selected AEs as signals out of 24 in the first example, and with 100 selected AEs as signals out of 1401 in the second example. Lastly, datasets are simulated with signals having heterogeneous η values using the (second) example of 100 selected signals out of 1401 AEs. This data has η_i as η for AEs of the selected 100 signals with marginal totals $\geq$ 2000, η_i as $2 \times \eta$ for AE signals with marginal totals between 500–2000, η_i as $3 \times \eta$ for those AE signals that have marginal totals between 100 and 500, and η_i as $15 \times \eta$ for AE signals with marginal totals less than 100 (see the η values in Table 3.2).

The effect of sample size is studied in a wide range (from 10 to 5000 including 2500 AEs, close to the observed sample size for the Montelukast example and 10 to 20,000 including 11,988 AEs, the observed sample size for the Heparin example). To understand the performance of the methods in the extreme case of sparse data, data are simulated with very small sample size (e.g., 10) to generate cell counts with a lot of zeroes.

3.2.2 Performance characteristics

Under each parameter configuration, 1000 datasets are simulated using (3.7). The power is defined as $\frac{\#\text{of times rejecting the null hypothesis}}{1000}$. The expression for power becomes type-I error rate when the data are simulated under the null hypothesis with all rr values as 1. The null hypothesis is rejected when there is at least one signal detected.

Sensitivity (ST), the proportion of actual positives which are correctly identified, is estimated by

$$\sum_L [\frac{\#\text{of signals correctly detected by the method in Lth simulated data}}{\text{total \# of true signals in the Lth simulated data}}]/1000.$$

We also estimate false discovery rate (FDR), the expected false positive rate, by

$$\sum_L [\frac{\#\text{of signals falsely detected by the method in the Lth simulated data}}{\text{total \# of detected signals in the Lth simulated data}}]/1000.$$

The values of ST and FDR are between 0 and 1. A method will have a good performance, if it has both a high ST value and a low FDR value. If data are simulated under the null hypothesis, the ST is not defined and FDR is equivalent to type-I error.

3.2.3 Simulation results

The simulation results including power, sensitivity, and FDR for different scenarios are presented in Tables 3.1 and 3.2.

Data with 24 AEs

The simulation based on the first example indicates that in case of a single signal, the power of all the methods increases when η, the marginal total for the selected signal, and the sample size increase. The power values for PRR are much higher than those for BCPNN and LRT; however, the type-I error for PRR is always high (0.5–0.7). For the simulated data with large sample size, or selected signal with large marginal total, the BCPNN method tends to provide good power values, but it also has a high type-I error rate (close to 0.3). For the data with small sample size (e.g., 10) and selected signal with low marginal total (e.g., 327), the BCPNN method has very poor power (lower than LRT method), and also very low type-I error (close to 0). The strength of the LRT method lies in the type-I error being close to 0.05 in all situations (with $\alpha = 0.05$). The power of LRT method increases and approaches to 1 when η, the marginal total for the selected signal, and the sample size become large.

The sensitivity (ST) of all three methods increases from 0 to 1 when the power increases from 0 to 1. However, FDR decreases when power increases. The FDR values for the PRR method remain at a high level (ranging from 0.15 to 0.7), which indicates that even though the power and the sensitivity of PRR is high, between 15% to 70% of the detected signals are not true signals (false positive alarms). The FDR values from BCPNN method (0 to 0.3) are higher than those for the LRT method except for some extreme cases. For example, when the sample size is very small (such as 10), both the power and sensitivity for the BCPNN method are close to 0, and the FDR is close to 0. The FDR for LRT method is well controlled between 0 and 0.05 with α as 0.05 for all scenarios.

The performance of the LRT method with varying α (results not shown) indicates that the type-I error for LRT is controlled at selected α for all situations. The power and sensitivity are lower when α is small (such as 0.001), but increase and approach 1 when the true signal is stronger and the sample size is larger. FDR is always controlled between 0 and the selected α value.

When randomly selected five AEs are assigned the same elevated η values, as expected, higher power values are observed for all the methods in case of data with multiple signals, as compared to data with a single signal. The power, type-I error, and sensitivity are similar to those observed in a single signal study. The FDR for data with multiple signals is lower compared to data with single signal.

Data with 1401 AEs

Evaluation of the performance of the methods with selected parameter configurations for the large data with 1401 AEs indicates that the performance characteristics of the methods for this large data are similar to those for the small data with 24 AEs. The few differences are noted below.

For a sample size of 11,988 and a single signal with 570 or 2103 marginal total, the power values for PRR and BCPNN are always 1 as η for the true signals varies from 1.5 to 8; however, the type-I error is close to 100% for both methods. The power of the LRT method is lower compared with that of the PRR and BCPNN methods, but the type-I error is well controlled below 0.05 level for all situations. Although the FDR for PRR and BCPNN methods decreases slightly when the signal is stronger, it still remains very high (0.9 to 1).

For 100 signals (with heterogeneous η values among the true signals) out of the 1401 AEs (η for the true signals $>=$ 1.5 and sample size 11,988), the power is close to 1 for all methods. LRT maintains the type-I error as 0.05, but the type-I error is 1 for both the PRR and BCPNN methods. When η increases from 1.5 to 5, sensitivity values increase from 0.3 to 0.9 for the LRT method; from 0.7 to 1 for PRR method, and from 0.5 to 0.9 for BCPNN method. FDR values are below 0.05 in all cases for the LRT method; and when η increase from 1 to 5, FDR values decrease from 1 to 0.2 for PRR method, and from 1 to 0 for BCPNN method. As seen in Table 3.3, in some cases the BCPNN method may have higher sensitivity and reasonably low FDR, thereby be more efficient than the LRT method. In practice, we recommend applying several methods of signal detection and following up on signals detected by multiple methods.

For simulation with true signals (η as 2 or 3) and small sample size (such as 10), PRR has power 1, LRT has power 0.1–0.2, and BCPNN has power close to 0. All methods have sensitivity close to 0–0.1 for data with small sample size (sparse data).

3.3 Applications to FAERS Data

The data files in FAERS database contain available information related to each event including patient demographics, route of administration, drug/biologic information, Medical Dictionary for Regulatory Activities (MedDRA) terms, medical history, treatment indication, and therapy start dates and end dates. For signal detection, MedDRA terminology of Preferred Term (PT) is often used to identify the AES, such as Hypotension, Hemorrhage, Cardiac procedure complication, Death, Bacteremia, etc. The file for drug/biologic information also has verbatim drug names such as HEPARIN SODIUM INJ, HEPARIN, HEPARIN FLUSH, HEPARIN SODIUM, etc. However, since one drug can have many different verbatim names, the generic name of the drug (which refers to the unique chemical makeup of a drug) is used in studying the drug-event association.

After summarizing the data files, the FAERS safety data can be presented in a tabular form with, for example, AE as the row variable and drug as the column variable. The count in each cell ($n_{ij}, i = 1, ..., I, j = 1, ..., J$) is the number of reported cases for a particular drug-event combination. Although the FAERS data include cases reported to FDA from 1968, there is more interest in signals that appear in recent years. Therefore, in the application section, we focus on the cases reported to FAERS from 2004–2008 (i.e., the most recent five-year data at the time of analysis) for more than 4000 drugs and 10,000 AEs for an investigation of possible signals. For any particular event, the investigator may consider only primary suspect drugs (may not be reliable in the current system, but unique for each event), or both primary and secondary suspect drugs, or all suspect and concomitant drugs.

The methods described in Section 3.1 were applied to FDA FAERS data from the first quarter of 2004 to the last quarter of 2008.

3.3.1 Montelukast analysis

Montelukast Sodium is prescribed for the treatment of asthma, prevention of exercise-induced asthma, and Allergic Rhinitis. All cases reported to FDA during the study period are aggregated and AEs are selected for the analysis on the basis of their relationship with suicidal and mood related behavior. There are 24 suicidal behavior and mood change-related AEs reported against Montelukast (primary suspect). The total number of suicidal behavior and mood change-related cases reported is 104,060, of which 2456 are primarily associated with Montelukast. The purpose of this analysis is to identify the suicidal and mood change-related AEs with high reporting rates primarily associated with Montelukast. The data and the signals detected by all the methods are included in Table 3.4.

As shown in Table 3.4, there are 13 AEs detected as signals by PRR method (PRR as the statistic) and BCPNN method (IC measures as the statistic). The lower bounds of the 95% confidence intervals of PRR and IC measures are greater than 1 and 0, respectively for these 13 detected AEs. The LRT method indicates that there are nine AEs with higher relative reporting rates(p-values ≤ 0.05). MGPS found seven AEs as signals with EB05 greater than 2.

The 13 signals detected by PRR and BCPNN methods include the nine signals detected by LRT method, and the signals detected by LRT method include all seven signals detected by MGPS method. The two AEs detected by LRT as signals, but not by MGPS are Emotional disorder with relative reporting rate of 2.4 and self-injurious ideation with relative reporting rate of 2.9.

The simulation study shows that although PRR and BCPNN methods have higher power to detect the signals, the FDR is not controlled. Therefore, there may be several false positive signals among the 13 signal found by PRR and BCPNN methods, whereas LRT detects fewer signals but with well controlled type-I error and fewer false positive signals.

3.3.2 Heparin analysis

Heparin, a blood thinner, has been widely used as an injectable anticoagulant and has attracted the attention of medical doctors and officers in recent years [33, 93, 136]. All cases reported to FDA during the study period are aggregated and only those AEs with Heparin as the primary suspect (PS) drug are counted. The purpose of the analysis is to identify the AEs with unusually high reporting rates primarily associated with Heparin.

There are a total of 1401 AEs with at least one reported case associated with Heparin (primary suspect). A total of 11,988 (aggregating all the 1401

AEs) cases are reported for Heparin and the total number of cases for all drugs and all AEs is 3,243,052. The marginal totals for the 1401 AEs range from 1 to 61,824. LRT identified 116 signals (AEs) out of the 1401 AEs for Heparin (p-value smaller than 0.05), MGPS method found 121 signals ($EB05 > 2$), PRR method found 392 signals ($PRR025 > 1$), and BCPNN method found 207 signals ($IC025 > 0$). The most significant signal is Heparin-induced thrombocytopenia. LRT has well-controlled type-I error and FDR, but not PRR and BCPNN from the simulation for large data. Therefore, it is possible that many of the extra signals detected by PRR, BCPNN, and MGPS methods for Heparin analysis are false positive signals.

One hundred and seven common signals are detected by MGPS and LRT methods; 14 signals detected by MGPS are not detected by LRT method, and 9 signals detected by LRT are not detected by MGPS method. All signals detected by MGPS are also detected by BCPNN. However, BCPNN detected 86 additional signals compared with MGPS. The number of common signals detected by BCPNN and LRT methods is 115; only one signal (White clot in blood present) detected by LRT method is not detected by the BCPNN method, and 92 signals detected by BCPNN method are not detected by the LRT method. All signals detected by BCPNN, MGPS, and LRT are also detected by PRR method.

For illustration, the stratified analysis is also conducted on the Heparin data with LRT and MGPS methods. Gender has been stratified into three strata: male, female, and unknown. The percentage of missing values (i.e., the percentage of cases in the unknown stratum) was 4.3% in all the AE cases reported, and 8.6% in all Heparin primary associated cases. Other variables, such as age, have higher percentage of missing (more than 40% missing values in the total cases reported), and are not considered in the stratified analysis. Note that the overall reporting rate for Heparin is 0.0023 for Female, 0.0033 for Male and 0.0056 for unknown gender in this 2004–2008 data. Since the proportion of unknown gender is small in the Heparin data, analysis could also be conducted on data excluding cases with unknown gender.

After gender adjustment, 116 AEs and 122 AEs are detected by LRT and MGPS methods (details of MGPS method with and without adjustment are included in Chapter 2), respectively. Thus, the total numbers of signals detected with and without gender adjustment are almost the same. Most of the AEs detected by LRT stay as signals with or without gender adjustment; seven AEs, detected without gender adjustment, are no longer signals with gender adjustment; and other seven AEs, not detected without gender adjustment, are detected as signal with adjustment. For MGPS method, two signals, without gender adjustment, disappear with gender adjustment; and three AEs, not detected without adjustment, become signals with adjustment.

If a signal can be explained fully by the stratified variable, such as gender, the signal will disappear. For example, Medication error has a relative reporting rate of 2.1, p-value of 0.001 with LRT method, and EB05 value of 2.37 with MGPS method, without stratification. However, relative reporting rate is 1.12, p-value is 1 with LRT method, and EB05 value is 1.82 with MGPS method with stratification because the pattern of reporting rate for Medication error for the three general categories is consistent with the overall AE pattern for Heparin. The high rate of 2.1 for "Medication error" without stratification can be explained fully by the gender pattern, so it is not a signal after gender adjustment. "Polycythaemia vera" is an AE signal detected with stratification, but not a signal without stratification. It has relative reporting rate of 16.91 and p-value of 0.327 from LRT method without stratification, but relative reporting rate of 45.52 and p-value of 0.024 with stratification. The signals may not be explained by gender at all, or may be explained only partially by gender. Overall, gender had a minor effect on the signal detection for the AEs associated with Heparin.

3.4 Notes and Discussion

In this Chapter, we introduce the basic LRT method and conduct a comprehensive study of the basic LRT method and other methods, commonly used for drug-event association evaluation. In this case, the LRT method only searches for AE signals for a particular drug or drug signals for a particular AE in the whole FAERS database. It can be extended to identify AE signals for data with multiple drugs in a drug class or for similar treatment indications, and to explore the post-market safety databases that include large and complex information for other products, such as devices, vaccines, food, etc. All analyses in Applications (Section 3.3) have been done for 2004–08 data with only primary suspect drugs. One can also explore data with all suspect (primary and secondary) drugs, or all (suspect and concomitant) drugs, depending on the research interest.

As shown in the simulation study, the LRT method controls the type-I error rate and the FDR is always between 0 and α (a pre-specified level of significance). Therefore, if there are only limited resources available for further investigation, a small value of α such as 0.01 or 0.001 could be used. Even with a smaller value of α, the LRT method will still have good power to detect signals that correspond to large sample size, large marginal total, or high relative reporting rate. For the other methods (PRR, BCPNN, and MGPS) discussed in Chapter 2, one could choose the lower bound of statistics (such as PRR, IC, EBGM) to correspond to 90%, 95%, or 99% confidence intervals and the thresholds of 0, 1, 2, or 3 to alleviate the issues of inflation of type-I error and FDR. Also, published literature suggests using joint criteria such as a lower bound greater than 1 and cell counts (n_{ij}) greater than 2 (see, for example, Hauben et al., [68]). The performance of PRR method with the additional criterion of $n_{ij} > 2$ was explored (data and results not shown) in a small simulation study. As expected, the additional criteria resulted in reduced values of the type-I error and FDR for PRR method, especially for sparse data (e.g., data with total sample size of 10 and 100). Thus our limited results suggest that such modified signal detection criteria and choices may reduce the number of detected signals and in turn reduce the FDR. There are also other metric/threshold combinations for PRR, cell counts, and other statistics such as chi-square statistic [35, 14, 72]. However, they are ad-hoc and not model-based, so their performance in real-time data analyses is difficult to study and as a result their routine use in practice is hard to defend.

Stratified analysis for covariate adjustment can be carried out for age, reporting year, and other covariates of interest. When the number of covariates increases, the cell counts may become sparse, adversely affecting the performance characteristics of the various methods of signal detection including LRT, and the interpretation of the detected signals with covariates adjustment may become very complex. In addition, Nam et. al. [112] propose a logistic regression model that can be used to account for many possible confounders in the context of post-market vaccine safety. The statistic is constructed based on the likelihood ratio test [80] and the expected counts are calculated using a Binomial distribution with probability parameter modeled by logistic regression model to incorporate covariates. Specifically, instead of using Equation 3.4 to estimate E_{ij}, Nam et. al. propose that the expected value of n_{ij}, under H_0, is

$$E_{ij} = E_{H_0}(n_{ij}) = \sum_{k=1}^{n_{.j}} logit^{-1}(x_{jk}^T \beta_i),$$

where x_{jk} are the covariates for j^{th} Vaccine in k^{th} report.

In the simulation study, many methods of signal detection are not able to control the type-I error and false discovery rate well, and some are not able to detect any signals for small or sparse data. The proposed LRT method detects signals with reasonable power and sensitivity, controls overall type-I error rate, and has well-controlled false discovery rate. We have shown that the method works well for data with a large or moderate number of reported cases in safety surveillance.

Many of the post-market safety databases that collect spontaneously and voluntarily submitted data, are subject to over-reporting, under-reporting, incomplete information, replicated information, and other potential biases. For example, one subject can be recorded several times in the database because the associated AE cases could have been reported to different reporting resources without consistent identification; event dates may not be available for many reports (missing dates); patients may not report an event because of limited resource for reporting or lack of knowledge, etc. Another issue in analyzing this type of data is that many AE preferred terms (PT) in MedDRA dictionaries are conceptually (medically) similar or synonymous (but literally different). Every PT is treated as a unique AE or condition in the FAERS data. In spite of corrections of the inconsistency and errors in the data, one subject can still contribute to several drug-AE combination cells, which may lead to some degree of correlation among the cells. According to our best knowledge, all the methods used for disproportionality analysis do not overcome this issue. However, when we relax the independence assumption (Section 6.2.4), the logLR is not affected by the added correlation structure.

The statistical methods discussed in this chapter are tools to find possible signals in large post-market safety databases, and provide a smaller group of signals for further investigation. The final determination of the true signals which are clinically meaningful is based on a careful examination of the medical records.

3.5 Further Discussion Points

In an article entitled "An evaluation of statistical approaches to post marketing surveillance" [38], Ding et. al. have compared PRR, FDR-PRR, ROR, FDR-ROR, BCPNN, FDR-BCPNN, and LRT methods through intensive simulation studies using evaluation metrics containing power, sensitivity, FDR, specificity, precision, and negative predicted value (NPV). The authors have not included MGPS and FDR-MGPS methods in the formal simulation evaluation, mainly due to computational and convergence issues. However, these methods have been included in their example. The authors have discussed the MGPS and FDR-MGPS performance evaluation in their Discussion section.

In this book, we do not provide details of the FDR-based methods [17, 16] such as FDR-ROR, FDR-PRR, FDR-BCPNN, and FDR-MGPS. These FDR-based methods do not conduct the comparison of the lower bounds of confidence intervals versus a threshold. Instead, the FDR-based methods propose to make decisions based on FDR values that can be estimated for the PRR, ROR, BCPNN, and MGPS methods. Additional details about the FDR-based methods can also be found in Ding et al. [38].

The methods and associated criteria for signal detection included in the paper (Ding et al. [38]) are shown in Table 3.5. The authors have discussed the advantages and disadvantages of the different pharmacovigilance methods (See Table 3.1).

The authors have listed the following points in the discussion and recommendation section.

- The LRT method does not have computational difficulties. It explicitly and successfully controls the type-I error and FDR while maintaining power and sensitivity. It is highly specific and precise. LRT is the preferred method in almost all circumstances, including when premium is placed on controlling the trade-off of FDR/type-I error and sensitivity/power of detection. As clearly indicated in the simulation study, the performance of PRR, ROR, BCPNN, FDR-PRR, FDR-ROR, FDR-BCPNN, and LRT methods depends on a number of characteristics such as the estimated relative risk of an AE of interest, the count of reports of a drug under consideration that contain the AE of interest, and the amount of control of the FDR deemed acceptable.

- When the marginal total is less than or equal to 100 and the relative reporting proportion is small, BCPNN is equivalent in performance to LRT. However, when the marginal total of the AE of interest is greater than 100 and less than or equal to 1,000, BCPNN has higher sensitivity than LRT but also higher FDR rate. The FDR rate of BCPNN decreases as the relative reporting proportion increases and stabilizes around 0.12. The performance of LRT, however, increases considerably when the marginal total of the AE of interest and/or relative reporting proportion increase.
- The second best performer in terms of the metrics used is BCPNN and FDR-BCPNN. Simulation studies show that FDR-BCPNN can control the FDR and type-I error well but has a lower power and sensitivity than LRT. BCPNN performs equivalently with LRT in cases that correspond to small marginal totals and low relative reporting proportions.
- The PRR and ROR methods have very high type-I error and false discovery rate (FDR), even though they have usually high power. The FDR criterion-based methods, FDR-PRR, and FDR-ROR obtain lower FDR values and lower levels of significance than their traditional versions. In spite of improvement in the FDR rate, these methods still exhibit unacceptably high FDR. On the other hand, FDR-BCPNN controls FDR and the level of significance well, but exhibits lower power and sensitivity.
- The MGPS method controls FDR and type-I error well, but is very conservative with limitations. The gamma mixture prior distribution may not be appropriate for every dataset (manifested as non-convergence of the associated algorithm); the multiple parameters associated with this prior distribution provide flexibility that may be appropriate for some datasets but not for others. Additionally, the choice of initial values for the algorithm that estimates the parameters of the prior distribution seems to be important. Moreover, it is possible, to obtain non-convergence in a rather high number of simulated datasets (up to 20%) although usually this number is around 5%-10%. A recent R package, entitled "openEBGM" offers several alternatives for estimating prior parameters. Given that there is no guarantee of convergence of this algorithm, it is still possible not to obtain convergence.

The findings from Ding et al. [38] summarized above (including the performance of LRT, PRR, and BCPNN methods and convergence issue of MGPS method) are consistent with the findings from our simulation results in Section 3.2. In the end of their Discussion, the authors have recommended, in practice, the use of LRT and BCPNN/FDR-BCPNN methods for safety signal detection.

3.6 Tables

TABLE 3.1
Advantages and disadvantages of different pharmacovigilance methods adapted from Ding et al. 2020.

Method	Advantages	Disadvantages
LRT	easy to interpret explicit control of family-wise type-I error and FDR generally high power/sensitivity and always high precision easy to compute	does not perform well in very sparse data sets in terms of power and sensitivity
BCPNN and FDR-BCPNN	easy to interpret robust in the presence of missing data BCPNN performs relatively well on sparse datasets FDR-BCPNN controls FDR and type-I error	depends on thresholds (FDR-BCPNN overcomes this issue) issue of selecting prior distribution relatively high type-I error mild signal overdetection
PRR and FDR-PRR	easy to compute and interpret high detection power relatively high sensitivity	depends on thresholds (FDR-PRR overcomes this issue) standard error for this statistic can be very large high type-I error and FDR rate proven to overdetect signals
ROR and FDR-ROR	simple to calculate and interpret not affected by under reporting high detection power relatively high sensitivity	depends on thresholds (FDR-ROR overcomes this issue)s tandard error for this statistics can be very large high type-I error and FDR rate proven to overdetect signals
MGPS and FDR-MGPS	easy to interpret robust when the expected counts are small	depends on thresholds (FDR-MGPS overcomes this issue) issue of selecting prior distribution convergence issues lowest sensitivity/power among all studies methods

TABLE 3.2
Performance characteristics of PRR, BCPNN, and LRT methods from Montelukast simulation study.

Marginal total	Sample size $n_{.j}$	η	Power(%)			Sensitivity			FDR		
			PRR	BCPNN	LRT	PRR	BCPNN	LRT	PRR	BCPNN	LRT
Single signal with marginal total as 2108 or 327											
2108	10	3	67	3	6	0.12	0.02	0.02	0.59	0.02	0.04
2108	50	3	74	26	21	0.36	0.18	0.18	0.49	0.08	0.03
2108	200	3	95	90	71	0.89	0.89	0.71	0.29	0.08	0.02
2108	300	3	99	97	85	0.98	0.97	0.85	0.26	0.09	0.02
2108	600	3	100	100	99	1.00	1.00	0.99	0.22	0.10	0.02
2108	1200	3	100	100	100	1.00	1.00	1.00	0.19	0.09	0.02
2108	2500	3	100	100	100	1.00	1.00	1.00	0.15	0.08	0.01
2108	5000	3	100	100	100	1.00	1.00	1.00	0.15	0.08	0.01
2108	300	1	62	29	5	NA	NA	NA	0.62	0.29	0.06
2108	300	1.5	71	41	9	0.31	0.22	0.05	0.49	0.21	0.04
2108	300	2	85	67	28	0.71	0.58	0.25	0.36	0.16	0.04
2108	300	3	99	97	85	0.98	0.97	0.85	0.26	0.09	0.02
2108	300	4	100	100	99	1.00	1.00	0.99	0.23	0.08	0.01
2108	300	5	100	100	100	1.00	1.00	1.00	0.21	0.07	0.01
327	300	1	62	29	5	NA	NA	NA	0.62	0.29	0.05
327	300	1.5	65	32	7	0.17	0.06	0.02	0.54	0.27	0.05
327	300	2	70	36	10	0.29	0.12	0.05	0.50	0.26	0.05
327	300	3	81	49	20	0.54	0.31	0.16	0.44	0.22	0.05
327	300	4	89	65	36	0.73	0.53	0.32	0.39	0.20	0.04
327	300	5	93	77	54	0.84	0.69	0.52	0.35	0.17	0.04
327	10	1	67	1	5	NA	NA	NA	0.67	0.01	0.05
327	10	1.5	67	1	5	0.04	0.00	0.00	0.64	0.01	0.05
327	10	2	67	1	5	0.05	0.00	0.00	0.63	0.01	0.05
327	10	3	68	1	6	0.09	0.00	0.00	0.62	0.01	0.05
327	10	4	69	2	6	0.11	0.00	0.01	0.61	0.02	0.05
327	10	5	69	2	6	0.14	0.00	0.01	0.60	0.02	0.05
2108	10	1	67	1	5	NA	NA	NA	0.67	0.01	0.05
2108	300	1	62	29	5	NA	NA	NA	0.62	0.29	0.05
2108	1200	1	54	32	5	NA	NA	NA	0.54	0.32	0.05
2108	2500	1	50	33	5	NA	NA	NA	0.50	0.33	0.05
Multiple signals (five randomly selected signals with varying marginal totals)											
NA	10	3	85	14	17	0.20	0.03	0.03	0.23	0.00	0.01
NA	50	3	99	90	65	0.39	0.25	0.15	0.12	0.00	0.01
NA	200	3	100	100	100	0.65	0.58	0.46	0.04	0.01	0.00
NA	300	3	100	100	100	0.71	0.66	0.55	0.04	0.01	0.00
NA	600	3	100	100	100	0.84	0.80	0.70	0.02	0.00	0.00
NA	1200	3	100	100	100	0.94	0.91	0.84	0.01	0.00	0.00
NA	2500	3	100	100	100	0.98	0.97	0.93	0.00	0.00	0.00
NA	5000	3	100	100	100	1.00	1.00	0.99	0.00	0.00	0.00
NA	300	1	62	29	5	NA	NA	NA	0.62	0.29	0.05
NA	300	1.5	91	80	44	0.27	0.22	0.09	0.21	0.08	0.02
NA	300	2	100	100	97	0.52	0.47	0.32	0.09	0.03	0.01
NA	300	3	100	100	100	0.71	0.66	0.55	0.04	0.01	0.00
NA	300	4	100	100	100	0.78	0.74	0.64	0.02	0.00	0.00
NA	300	5	100	100	100	0.81	0.77	0.67	0.01	0.00	0.00

TABLE 3.3
Performance characteristics of PRR, BCPNN, and LRT methods from Heparin simulation study.

Marginal total	Sample size $n_{.j}$	η	Power(%)			Sensitivity			FDR		
			PRR	BCPNN	LRT	PRR	BCPNN	LRT	PRR	BCPNN	LRT
Single signal with marginal total as 2103 or 570											
2103	10	3	100	0	5	0.02	0.00	0.00	1.00	0.00	0.05
2103	100	3	100	46	5	0.18	0.00	0.00	0.99	0.46	0.05
2103	1000	3	100	100	7	0.32	0.14	0.03	0.99	0.98	0.05
2103	3000	3	100	100	12	0.73	0.57	0.08	0.99	0.95	0.05
2103	8000	3	100	100	45	0.94	0.91	0.42	0.98	0.95	0.04
2103	11988	3	100	100	72	0.98	0.98	0.70	0.98	0.95	0.04
2103	20000	3	100	100	97	1.00	1.00	0.97	0.98	0.95	0.02
2103	11988	1	100	100	5	0.02	0.02	0.00	1.00	1.00	0.05
2103	11988	1.5	100	100	5	0.27	0.27	0.00	0.99	0.99	0.05
2103	11988	2	100	100	16	0.71	0.71	0.12	0.99	0.96	0.04
2103	11988	3	100	100	72	0.98	0.98	0.70	0.98	0.95	0.04
2103	11988	4	100	100	97	1.00	1.00	0.97	0.98	0.95	0.03
2103	11988	5	100	100	100	1.00	1.00	1.00	0.98	0.95	0.02
2103	11988	8	100	100	100	1.00	1.00	1.00	0.98	0.95	0.02
570	11988	1	100	100	5	0.02	0.02	0.00	1.00	1.00	0.05
570	11988	1.5	100	100	5	0.10	0.10	0.00	1.00	0.99	0.05
570	11988	2	100	100	7	0.26	0.26	0.01	1.00	0.99	0.06
570	11988	3	100	100	16	0.63	0.63	0.12	0.99	0.97	0.04
570	11988	4	100	100	40	0.86	0.86	0.36	0.98	0.96	0.05
570	11988	5	100	100	63	0.94	0.94	0.61	0.98	0.95	0.04
570	11988	8	100	100	96	1.00	1.00	0.96	0.98	0.95	0.02
Randomly selected 100 signals with homogeneous η											
NA	11988	1	100	100	5	NA	NA	NA	1.00	1.00	0.05
NA	11988	1.5	100	100	98	0.26	0.20	0.03	0.61	0.40	0.01
NA	11988	2	100	100	100	0.43	0.35	0.15	0.45	0.22	0.00
NA	11988	3	100	100	100	0.57	0.48	0.30	0.32	0.11	0.00
NA	11988	4	100	100	100	0.65	0.54	0.38	0.25	0.07	0.00
NA	11988	5	100	100	100	0.70	0.58	0.44	0.21	0.04	0.00
Randomly selected 100 signals with inhomogeneous η											
NA	11988	1	100	100	5	0.39	0.24	0.07	0.53	0.39	0.01
NA	11988	1.5	100	100	100	0.71	0.56	0.21	0.34	0.17	0.00
NA	11988	2	100	100	100	0.87	0.76	0.45	0.27	0.10	0.00
NA	11988	3	100	100	100	0.95	0.88	0.73	0.20	0.05	0.00
NA	11988	4	100	100	100	0.97	0.92	0.84	0.17	0.03	0.00
NA	11988	5	100	100	100	0.98	0.94	0.88	0.14	0.02	0.00
NA	10	3	100	1	17	0.02	0.00	0.00	0.76	0.00	0.04
NA	100	3	100	72	20	0.11	0.01	0.00	0.71	0.18	0.02
NA	1000	3	100	100	100	0.44	0.19	0.05	0.45	0.12	0.00
NA	2000	3	100	100	100	0.63	0.35	0.14	0.36	0.10	0.00
NA	3000	3	100	100	100	0.73	0.48	0.24	0.31	0.08	0.00
NA	8000	3	100	100	100	0.90	0.78	0.59	0.23	0.06	0.00
NA	11988	3	100	100	100	0.95	0.88	0.73	0.20	0.05	0.00
NA	20000	3	100	100	100	0.98	0.94	0.87	0.17	0.05	0.00

TABLE 3.4

Suicidal and mood alteration-related signals (AEs) detected for Montelukast in the FAERS data with cases reported to FDA during 2004–2008.

AE	marginal total		n_{ij}		RR		PRR025		IC025		LLR (p-value)		EB05	
	ps	alls	ps	alls	ps	alls	ps	alls	ps	alls	ps	alls	ps	alls
Abnormal behavior	6847	8817	329	331	2.74	2.35	2.0	2.4	0.9	0.9	72.8 (0.001)	85.05(0.001)	2.48	2.68
Anhedonia	963	1179	12	12	0.74	0.59	0.3	0.3	-1.7	-1.5	0.0	0.0	0.44	0.47
Anxiety	21267	26287	276	278	0.81	0.56	0.4	0.5	-1.0	-0.9	0.0	0.0	0.73	0.73
Completed suicide	10106	21856	49	56	0.31	0.13	0.1	0.1	-2.7	-3.1	0.0	0.0	0.25	0.27
Crying	4469	5413	162	165	2.38	1.82	1.3	1.6	0.4	0.6	13.7 (0.001)	23.2(0.001)	2.06	1.95
Decreased interest	406	465	17	17	2.49	2.12	1.1	1.3	0.1	0.4	2.3	3.8	1.45	1.63
Depressed mood	2510	3110	69	69	1.72	1.29	0.9	1.0	-0.1	0.0	0.8	2.0	1.37	1.36
Depression	24025	30449	451	456	1.16	0.84	0.7	0.8	-0.5	-0.4	0.0	0.0	1.08	1.08
Depressive symptom	245	355	3	3	0.77	0.49	0.2	0.1	-2.2	-2.3	0.0	0.0	0.27	0.26
Dysphoria	255	378	1	1	0.24	0.15	0.0	0.0	-3.8	-3.9	0.0	0.0	0.06	0.06
Emotional disorder	2108	2544	82	84	2.43	1.94	1.3	1.6	0.4	0.6	8.9 (0.002)	14.6(0.001)	1.96	1.99
Emotional distress	3137	3803	8	8	0.15	0.12	0.1	0.1	-4.0	-3.8	0.0	0.0	0.09	0.09
Feeling guilty	100	133	2	2	1.19	0.87	0.2	0.2	-1.8	-1.8	0.0	0.0	0.28	0.28
Feeling of despair	422	517	18	18	2.67	2.02	1.2	1.3	0.1	0.3	2.6	3.6	1.56	1.56
Frustration	333	402	16	16	3.05	2.21	1.3	1.4	0.2	0.4	3.2	4.3(0.043)	1.68	1.68
Intentional self-i	1227	1642	44	45	2.14	1.60	1.1	1.2	0.2	0.2	3.4	4.2	1.59	1.69
Mood altered	2279	2751	129	129	3.53	2.81	2.1	2.4	1.0	1.2	38.8 (0.001)	48.6(0.001)	2.96	2.90
Mood swings	3294	3811	166	165	3.14	2.61	1.9	2.2	0.9	1.1	39.3 (0.001)	54.4(0.001)	2.70	2.64
Negative thoughts	161	183	12	12	4.65	3.80	1.8	2.2	0.6	0.8	5.6 (0.009)	7.2(0.003)	2.03	2.04
Self-injurious ide	579	736	27	27	2.85	2.13	1.4	1.5	0.4	0.5	5.1 (0.016)	6.1(0.009)	1.86	1.91
Suicidal behavior	327	424	27	27	5.00	3.71	2.5	2.6	1.1	1.2	14.6 (0.001)	15.6(0.001)	3.02	3.17
Suicidal ideation	10807	13406	433	433	2.45	2.05	1.7	1.9	0.6	0.7	59.2 (0.001)	78.6(0.001)	2.25	2.27
Suicide attempt	7604	13813	115	116	0.94	0.46	0.5	0.4	-0.9	-1.3	0.0	0.0	0.80	0.80
Tearfulness	589	737	7	7	0.79	0.55	0.2	0.3	-1.9	-1.8	0.0	0.0	0.40	0.37
Total signals detected	NA	NA	NA	NA	NA	NA	13	14	13	14	9	10	7	6

RR rate is relative reporting rate. ps indicates primary suspect analysis and alls indicates all suspect (primary and secondary) analysis. PRR025 is the lower bound of 95% CI for PRR (PRR method), IC025 is the lower bound of 95% CI for IC (BCPNN method), EB05 is the 90% CI for EBGM (MGPS method), and LLR is the statistic from LRT method. Only p-values less than 0.05 for LRT method are presented in the table.

TABLE 3.5

Methods of signal detection and associated criteria for signal detection adapted from Ding et al. 2020.

Method	Index used in simulation and empirical analysis	Criteria for signal detection
PRR	PRR	Lower bound of the 95% CI of $PRR > 1$
	FDR-PRR	FDR value of corresponding PT-drug combination < 0.025
ROR	ROR	Lower bound of the 95% CI of $ROR > 1$
	FDR-ROR	FDR value of corresponding PT-drug combination < 0.025
MGPS	MGPS	the test statistics $EB05 > 2$
	FDR-MGPS	the modified FDR-MGPS test statistic with cutoff value $\alpha = 0.05$
BCPNN	BCPNN	The test statistic IC025, i.e., the lower bound of 95% CI of $IC > 0$
	FDR-BCPNN	The modified FDR-BCPNN test statistic with cutoff value $\alpha = 0.025$
LRT	LRT	p-value< 0.05

4

LRT Methods for Drug Classes

In Chapter 3, the basic LRT method was applied to the FAERS data reported during 2004–2008 including thousands of drugs for illustration. In this chapter, we present the use of the basic LRT method for signal detection to a subset of data including only a few drugs within a drug class of interest from the entire FAERS database [79]. Note that the expected counts of the drug-AE combinations in the data including drugs within a drug class are not the same as those obtained from the large data that includes all drugs.

In addition, an extended LRT method using double maximum procedure [149] is presented to detect signals for certain drug classes (in Section 4.2) and a modified LRT method with weight matrix [79] is discussed for the detection of signals including a single drug or drug combinations in the entire FAERS data (in Section 4.3). Conversely, this modified LRT method can also be used for detecting signals including a single AE or AE combinations (if AEs belong to one AE group such as System Organ Class (SOC)).

For comparison, some methods described in Chapter 2 (such as PRR, sB.5 (sB method with $c = 0.5$), sB.01 (sB method with $c = 0.01$), sB.0001 (sB method with $c = 0.0001$), and BCPNN) are applied to data for the detection of signals including a single drug/AE.

4.1 Signals for Drug Class

4.1.1 Drug signals in FAERS data

Here, signals of single drug-AE combination are defined as the signals including a single drug for a fixed AE of interest or a single AE for a fixed drug of interest. For example, GBCA 1 (a single drug) can be a drug signal for fibrosis and sneezing (a single AE) can be an AE signal for drug GBCA 2.

GBCA 1, GBCA 2, ..., and GBCA 5 are five drugs in a gadolinium-based contrast agent drug class for diagnostic imaging procedures to enhance the quality of magnetic resonance imaging (MRI). The year of first approval of the five drugs ranges from 1988 to 2004. The exploration of the five-year data (2005–2009, one year after the last approval) including all the drugs and AEs from FAERS is presented in this section. The total reported drug-event combination counts for GBCA 1, GBCA 2, GBCA 3, GBCA 4, and GBCA 5 are 9596, 1953, 4213, 2309, and 3743 in the five-year period (2005–2009), respectively.

The results of using basic LRT and other methods for the five year data including all the drugs and AEs are shown in Table 4.1. For example, for the period 2005–09, and GBCA 1 as the drug, the total number of AE (PT) names (reported with cases associated with GBCA 1) is 998, and the number of AE signals (single AE term such as NSF) detected from PRR, sB.5, sB.01, sB.0001, BCPNN, and LRT are 296, 102, 130, 141, 154, and 91, respectively.

The sB.01 and sB.0001 provide similar number of signals, but sB.5 identifies fewer number of signals. Except PRR (most sensitive, but with many false-positive signals), BCPNN typically detects more number of signals than those by sB methods. The signals detected by the LRT method are usually fewer than those detected by sB.5 methods. Among GBCAs, GBCA 1 appears to have more number of AE signals detected, while the other four GBCAs have similar number of signals detected.

Top signals detected by LRT method, in the order of the values of the statistic "maxlogLR" (higher value, more significant), are presented in Table 4.1. For example, for GBCA 1, the first AE (NSF) corresponding to order No. 1 with a RR of 191, is the most significant signal, followed by Urticaria, Sneezing, Fibrosis, Skin fibrosis, etc.

All five GBCAs have NSF as the most significant signal. The RRs are all high (in hundreds). Among the five GBCAs, GBCA 3 has the highest relative reporting rate for NSF (826 for 2005-09). Other signals (with some as PT terms related to NSF) include fibrosis, skin fibrosis, scar, skin tightness, etc.

4.1.2 Signals of single drug-AE combination

The safety signals for drug GBCA1 are explored using the data with only drugs within the GBCA drug class (not the entire FAERS data including all drugs). The signals detected in this subsection are not the signals in the FAERS data, but the signals within the subset of FAERS database including only the drugs in a given drug class (e.g., gadolinium drug class). An AE signal for all GBCA drugs in the FAERS data analysis, may not appear as a signal within the drug class data analysis because the proportion of one drug among all the drugs $n_{i.}/n_{..}$ and the expected value of event counts assuming equal reporting rate $n_{.j} \times \frac{n_{i.}}{n_{..}}$ are different in the two types of data.

The number of signals detected by PRR, sB methods, BCPNN, and LRT methods are shown in Table 4.2. Since sB.01 and sB.0001 have similar results, the results for sB.0001 are not included in Table 4.2. PRR detects a large number of signals, many of which are likely to be false positive. More often, sB.5 detects fewer signals than BCPNN and LRT. In this application, the BCPNN method is more sensitive than sB methods and LRT method.

Prospectively, the signals can be evaluated for 2005, 2005–2006, 2005–2007, 2005–2008, and 2005–2009 assuming that the researcher starts the study with only 2005 data and monitors the signals over time. Because of the limited space, only the results for 2005, 2005–07, and 2005–09 data are included in Table 4.2. For the first year 2005, almost all methods, except PRR, do not identify any signals. For the 2nd cumulative period (2005–06) and the 3rd cumulative period (2005–07), some signals are identified by all methods. Additional signals are detected in the last cumulative period (2005–2009).

PRR, BCPNN, and LRT methods, but not the sB method, detected more signals in GBCA 1 than the other GBCAs within the drug class.

The top signals for the drugs in gadolinium class obtained by the LRT method are shown in Table 4.3. NSF, as an AE for all the GBCA drugs in the FAERS data (described in last section), is no longer a signal for every drug when the data only includes drugs within the gadolinium drug class. Prospectively, we show the signals detected from 2005, 2005–2006, ..., and 2005–09. There are no signals for GBCA 1 from 2005, 2005–06, and 2005–07. Urticaria and Dyspnea become the top two signals starting from the 4th cumulative period (2005–08). For GBCA 3, NSF starts being identified as a signal from the 2005–06 period with relative reporting rates decreasing from 8 to 3 over the years, and Hemodialysis becomes a signal from the 2005–08 period with RR of 5 within the drug class. "Off label use" only becomes a signal for GBCA 4 in the 5th cumulative data 2005–09 with RR of 6. GBCA 5 has Nausea as a signal from the 1st period (year 2005) and Hypersensitivity becomes a signal from the cumulative period 2005–06, with RR values ranging from 2.8 to 4.9.

4.1.3 Performance evaluation using simulation

Statistically, as method's performance can be evaluated in terms of power, sensitivity, and false discovery rate (FDR) with simulated data generated using information (such as marginal totals) from the real data. A high power and low FDR increases confidence in the detected signals from the real data. The high power and sensitivity indicate that very few potential signals were missed in the real data. A simulation study conducted to illustrate the validation of the GBCA 5 AE signals using data including only the gadolinium drugs during different cumulative periods is discussed below.

Data are simulated with several AE signals for GCBA 5. The marginal row total counts $(n_{1.}, \cdots, n_{I.})$ and the sample size $(n_{.j})$ information are obtained from real data for the time periods discussed in the above application. Five AE signals were identified for GBCA 5: Hypersensitivity, Nausea, Vomiting, Anaphylactoid reaction, and Retching. For each situation (shown in Table 4.4), 1000 datasets are simulated using Equation 3.7 described in Chapter 3. The η values for the five GBCA 5-AE combinations compared to the gadolinium drug class range from 2 to 5. In the simulation study, these five AEs were assigned a η value of greater than 1 (e.g., $\eta = 1.5, 2, 3, 5, 10$) for alternative data. All other GBCA 5-AE combinations were assigned η as 1. For null data generation, $\eta = 1$ for all AEs indicates that the relative reporting rate for all the AEs is 1.

The power, sensitivity, and FDR are defined in Chapter 3 (Section 3.2.2). The simulation results show that, in general, the performance pattern of the different methods for different choices of the η values are similar: higher values of power and sensitivity along with lower values of FDR are associated with higher η values. Therefore, only the results for η of 1, 2, and 3, are shown in Table 4.4. Note that when true signals are given η of 1, there are no signal in the data. The type-I error is evaluated instead of power. Sensitivity is not defined and FDR is the type-I error. For year 2005 (i.e., beginning of the study periods), PRR, BCPNN, and LRT have moderate or good powers, but sB.5 and sB.01 do not have the requisite power to identify at least one signal for GBCA 5 till the study reaches three- or four-year cumulative data (2005–08). With higher RR (e.g., 5 or above), all methods have requisite power even for the one year (2005) data.

PRR method has very high sensitivity, but also very high FDR for all study periods. BCPNN method also has relatively high sensitivity for all study periods, but low FDR for early study periods (2005, 2005–06, 2005–07). However, when RR=2, BCPNN method has higher FDR rates 0.12 and 0.23 for cumulative data periods 2005–08 and 2005–09 (later periods), respectively. sB.5 and sB.01 have high sensitivity and low FDR when the power is high (e.g., for the last two or three cumulative periods), but may not catch the signals in early periods (delay in detection). LRT has high power, moderate sensitivity, and very low FDR for all study periods and RR values. For LRT, the signals detected in the application have a high chance of being the true signals, and for all the periods.

4.2 Ext-LRT Signal Detection using Double Maximum

Zhao et al. [149] proposed an extended LRT method (Ext-LRT) for detection of drug-AE signals within a certain drug class using the FAERS data. The signals detected by basic LRT in Section 4.1.1 are drug-AE signals for a fixed GBCA drug using data including only drugs within the BGCA drug class.

4.2.1 Ext-LRT statistic and statistical inference

The authors [149] assume that the drug class has J different drugs (usually J is a small number), and for the jth drug, the number of reports for ith AE and all other AEs (excluding ith AE) have independent Poisson distributions :

$$n_{ij} \sim Poisson(n_{i.}p_{ij});$$
$$n_{.j} - n_{ij} \sim Poisson((n_{..} - n_{i.})q_{ij}),$$

where p_{ij} is the reporting rate of the jth drug for ith AE, and q_{ij} is the reporting rate of the jth drug for all the other AEs, excluding ith AE.

The null and alternative hypotheses for detecting AE signal in drug j are, H_{0j}: $p_{ij} = q_{ij} = p_{0j}$ for all AEs in drug j versus H_{aj}: $p_{ij} > q_{ij}$ for at least one AE.

The likelihood ratio for ith AE in jth drug as:

$$LR_{ij} = \frac{L_a(\hat{p}_{ij}, \hat{q}_{ij})}{L_0(\hat{p}_{j0})} = \left(\frac{n_{ij}}{E_{ij}}\right)^{n_{ij}} \left(\frac{n_{.j} - n_{ij}}{n_{.j} - E_{ij}}\right)^{n_{.j} - n_{ij}}$$

and the LRT test statistic for testing H_{0j} versus H_{aj} for at least one AE, is $MLR_j = max_i(LR_{ij})$,$i = 1, \ldots I$. The test statistic for testing the global null H_0 versus the global alternative H_a is

$$MMLR = max_j(MLR_j) = max_j(max_i(LR_{ij}I(\hat{p}_{ij} > \hat{q}_{ij}))),$$

where maximum is taken over $i = 1, \ldots I$ and $j = 1, \ldots J$.

The Ext-LRT can also be used to perform stratified analysis where there are a small number of covariates present such as age and gender. If there are S strata, the expected counts in s_{th} stratum can be calculated using

$$E_{ij}^{(s)} = \frac{n_{i.}^{(s)} n_{.j}^{(s)}}{n_{..}^{(s)}}$$

and then LR_{ij} can be computed using $E_{ij} = \sum_s E_{ij}^{(s)}$.

For the empirical distribution of MLR under H_0, we still apply the Monte Carlo simulation approach defined above to all the J drugs in the drug class. For each drug j in the drug class under H_0 we generate 999 datasets using conditional Multinomial distribution:

$$(n_{1j}, n_{2j}, \ldots, n_{Ij})|n_{.j}; n_{i.}, \ldots, n_{I.} \sim Multinomial\left(n_{.j}, \left(\frac{n_{1.}}{n_{..}}, \ldots, \frac{n_{I.}}{n_{..}}\right)\right), \tag{4.1}$$

and compute 1000 values of MLR including the one from the real data, for $j = 1, \ldots, J$. This results into $1000 \times J$ MLR values. The null hypothesis is rejected at $\alpha = 0.05$ level if the value of MLR from the observed dataset is greater than the $(1 - \alpha)$th percentile of the $1000 \times J$ MLR values T_α.

After AE associated with the largest LR_{ij} is identified as signal ($LR_{ij} > T_\alpha$), we move to the AE with the second largest value of LR_{ij}, determine if it is a signal, and so on. This way, like LRT, the Ext-LRT method also controls the type-I error.

We can show that MLR also controls the FDR. If V is the random variable denoting the number of false signals, and S is the random variable denoting the number of the true signals detected, then FDR is defined as $E(\frac{V}{V+S}|H_0)$.

In using the Ext-LRT for a drug class, the cutoff value T_α is the $100(1-\alpha)$

percentile point of $max_j(max_i(LR_{ij}))$, which is greater than or equal to T_{α_j} for each j. Thus,

$$E(FDR) = E\left(\frac{V}{V+S}|H_0\right) = \sum_{j=1}^{J} P(drug_j)E\left(\frac{V}{V+S}|H_0, drug_j\right)$$
$$= \frac{1}{J}\sum_{j=1}^{J} E\left(\frac{V}{V+S}|H_{0j}\right) \leq \frac{1}{J}\sum_{j=1}^{J} \alpha = \alpha,$$

where the last inequality follows from Ref. [80]. Hence, FDR is controlled under α for the Ext-LRT.

4.2.2 Application of Ext-LRT method

Table 4.5 shows the signal detection results from applying the LRT and Ext-LRT methods to the "gadolinium-based contrast agents" (GBCAs). The authors [149] select five GBCAs in the drug class, labeled as GBCA1, GBCA2, GBCA3, GBCA4, and GBCA5 (not in any specific order), to mask their names, using the FAERS 2009-2013 dataset. $I = 1,804$ PTs associated with GBCAs have been reported.

The number of signals detected within GBCAs drug class using the methods of LRT and Ext-LRT are listed in Table 4.5. Applying the LRT method to each of the five drugs in the drug class results in the detection of 115, 71, 70, 73, and 80 signals for the five GBCA drugs, respectively; whereas with the Ext-LRT, 107, 65, 68, 71, and 78 signals are detected, respectively. Ext-LRT detects fewer signals than LRT across the five drugs.

Cross-checking the signals in the five GBCAs drugs results in 20 common signals being detected within this drug class. The top signals from Ext-LRT are listed in Table 4.6, and Nephrogenic systemic fibrosis (NSF), fibrosis, skin hypertrophy, skin induration, skin tightness, skin fibrosis and scar are the strongest signals for this Gadolinium class. All signals detected by Ext-LRT for each drug are contained in the signals detected by LRT. Furthermore, the orders of the signals detected by these two methods are the same.

The observed percentages of true zeros are big ($> 90\%$) listed in Table 4.5. Another method for handling data with large zeros is discussed in detail in Chapter 5.

4.3 LRT for Identification of Signals Using Weight Matrix

In Sections 4.1 and 4.2, LRT method is used for data including only drugs within a drug class for AE signal detection. In the illustrations, the drug is the column variable and AE is the row variable (there are a total of I AEs and J drugs). As presented in this section, the LRT method [79] is modified for identifying signals including not only single drug or AE but also several drugs in one drug class (collection of drugs for same indication) or several medically/biologically related AEs (collection of AEs), by incorporating a weight matrix for the drugs (or AEs) of interest.

The weight matrix can be constructed using the drug class information (for example, a weight of 1 for drugs within a drug class, and 0 for drugs not in the particular drug class), or using the dose information (a weight of 1 for drugs with similar doses, and 0 for drugs with different doses), and other information (such as toxicity and chemical structure of the drugs). The drug class could be the class of drugs for similar indication, with similar chemical structure, or just a class of drugs depending on the interest of the researchers. For example, the drugs in Gadolinium drug class have similar chemical structure and all are contrast agents for medical imaging. The AE group could be AEs associated with one organ (system organ class: SOC), high-level group terms (HLGT), high-level terms (HLT) defined by Medical Dictionary for Regulatory Activities (MedDRA), or just a group of AEs of interest. The individual drugs in a drug class or individual AEs related to the same system can have similar signal patterns, and the collection of multiple drugs and AEs may lead to stronger signals as a whole.

We use this method for the drugs in the gadolinium drug class and in Statin drug class for one AE of interest (multiple AEs of interest are shown in the later section). Similar application of FAERS can be conducted for a group of AEs (for a fixed drug of interest). For example, Preferred Terms (PTS) such as sleep terror, screaming, morbid thoughts, educational problem, aggression, mood alternations, abnormal behavior, nightmare, etc., that are all related to mental problem (a group of AEs); PTs such as acute hepatic failure, ALT abnormal, Ascites, Blood bilirubin abnormal, Cholestatic liver injury, Hepatic atrophy, Hepatomegaly, Reye's syndrome, etc., that are all related to Hepatocellular injury.

4.3.1 Modified LRT statistic and statistical inference

The basic LRT method described in Chapter 3 is modified to identify drug collection signals for a fixed AE of interest. Although this section focuses on drug classes, the method can also be used for AE groups. In the large $I \times J$ matrix described in Chapter 3, the column variable is AE and the row variable is drug. A $I \times I$ weight matrix is defined as $w(i,i^*) \equiv w_{ii^*} = 1(i \geq i^*)$, if ith and i*th rows (drugs) are in the same drug class, and $w_{i,i^*} = 0$ if ith and i*th rows (drugs) are not known to be in the same drug class. I is the total number of rows (single drugs) in the large $I \times J$ data matrix including AE reports. Note that if the relationship between the ith and i*th rows is unknown (i.e., if they are not presumed to be in the same class), we define $w_{ii^*} = 0(i \neq i^*)$. The matrix $w(i,i^*)$ of weights is to be defined only for the diagonal and upper diagonal elements as the lower diagonal elements can be defined by symmetry, $w_{ii^*} = w_{i^*i}$.

Let g represent a collection that could include a single drug or multiple drugs (if in one class) according to the weight matrix. Let H be the total number of g's (collection of drugs). Clearly, $H > I$. Let $g_1 = \{1\}, \cdots, g_I = \{I\}$ represent the collections with size 1 (i.e., all the I single drugs). For g_h with size 2 or more ($h = I+1, \cdots, H$), one can start from the first row of the $I \times I$ weight matrix, and identify all the combinations (with size of 2 to a pre-specified maximum size of the drug classes) of the drugs that have value 1 in the cell for each row. Because of the symmetric feature of the weight matrix, the g-collections with size >= 2 can be obtained using the upper right triangle above the diagonal line.

For example, as shown in Figure 4.1, consider a total of four drugs (I=4), and suppose that Drugs 1, 2, and 4 belong to one drug class, and Drug 3 belongs to another drug class. The 4×4 weight matrix is constructed in the table and one circle represents one g. For g-collections with size 1, $g_1 = 1$ can represent drug 1, and $g_4 = 4$ can represent drug 4. For collection size >= 2 from the upper triangle part, possible combinations for the first row are $g_5 = \{1,2\}, g_6 = \{1,4\}, g_7 = \{1,2,4\}$; possible combinations for the 2nd row are $g_8 = \{2,4\}$; possible combinations for the 3rd row are none, and possible combinations for the 4th row are none.

The possible signals are any of the g-collections. The $logLR$ described in Chapter 3 can be calculated for each g. Let $n_{g_h j} = \sum_{i \in g_h} n_{ij}$ be the number of reported counts for the g_hth collection and jth column, and $n_{g_h .}$ be the marginal total of counts for the g_hth group (sum of the marginal totals for the drugs included in g_h). Note that if the exposure information is available for each drug or AE, then the $n_{g_h .}$ is the sum of the exposure from all drugs in the collection g_h.

The likelihood ratio for (g_h, j)th collection-column combination is then

$$LR_{g_h j} = \frac{\max L_a}{\max L_0} = \frac{L_a(\hat{p},\hat{q})}{L_0(\hat{p}*)} = (\frac{n_{g_h j}}{E_{g_h j}})^{n_{g_h j}} (\frac{n_{.j} - n_{g_h j}}{n_{.j} - E_{g_h j}})^{n_{.j} - n_{g_h j}},$$

where $E_{g_h j} = \frac{n_{g_h .} \times n_{.j}}{n_{..}}$, $n_{.j} = \sum_{i=1}^{I} n_{ij}, n_{i.} = \sum_{j=1}^{J} n_{ij}, n_{..} = \sum_{i=1}^{I} n_{i.}, h = 1, \cdots, H$. For a fixed column $j = j*$ (AE_{j^*}), the test statistic is then defined as maximum log likelihood ratios over the H groups:

$$maxLLR = \max_{g_h} logLR_{g_h j*}, h = 1, \cdots, H.$$

Searching for signals of a particular AE of interest among the g-collections in a large database may require recording of the drugs by drug class (drugs in the same drug class will have adjacent order number) to save time for computation. The maximum size of the g (covering one drug or multiple drugs) can be restricted as the maximum number of drugs in the known drug classes (e.g., 3, 5, 8, or 10) in a study. The possible collections of g include the I single drugs plus the combinations of the drugs belonging to the pre-specified drug classes according to the weight matrix. In Figure 4.1, the maximum size of the g-collections is 3.

As discussed in Chapter 3, the distribution of MLLR under H_0 is not analytically tractable and can be obtained using Monte Carlo (MC) simulation. For each MC data, the $n_{1j*}, \cdots, n_{Ij*}$ can be generated through the same way as described in Chapter 3 (Equation 3.2). For each simulated null data, once the $n_{1j*}, \cdots, n_{Ij*}$ are generated, the $n_{g_h j*} = \sum_{i \in g_h} n_{ij*}$ with $h > I$ for g_h with collection size ≥ 2.

The MaxLLR (max of logLR over g_h) can be obtained for each MC data. The LLR_{g_h} (in the observed data) can be ordered from largest to smallest and the LLR_{g_h} can be compared with the MaxLLR value from MC simulation. If the hth collection in the observed data has $LLR_{g_h} >$ the 95th percentile of the 10000 MaxLLR from the null data (*threshold*), then the g_h is a signal. One can also evaluate the g_h with the 2nd largest LLR_{g_h} value, the 3rd largest LLR_{g_h} value, and declare them as signals if $LLR_{g_h} >$ *threshold*. This modified LRT method has the same feature as that of basic LRT method in terms of type-I error and false discovery rate control.

4.3.2 Applications in detection of signals — Collection of drugs

In order to search for a single drug signal and drug collection signals for a fixed AE of interest, the modified LRT method incorporating weight matrix is applied to FAERS 2005–09 data including a total of 4273 drugs (suspect drugs only).

The purpose is to search for drugs or drug combinations with higher relative reporting rates for a particular AE of interest. Several AEs are selected for exploration, such as NSF, Fibrosis, Hypersensitivity, Hemodialysis, Myalgia, Rhabdomyolysis, and increase in Blood creatinine (CPK). For each AE of interest, a total of 4273 drugs are compared in the FAERS data, and the LRT method detects the signals including a single drug or several drugs that belonging to one drug class.

For illustration, define $w_{ii^*} = 1$ for the five drugs (GBCA 1, GBCA 2, GBCA 3, GBCA 4, and GBCA 5) within the gadolinium drug class and the six drugs (Atorvastatin, Fluvastatin, Lovastatin, Pravastatin, Rosuvastatin, and Simvastatin) within the Statins respectively, and $w_{i,i^*} = 0$ for other drugs (generic names) in the weight matrix. One can also add any additional information on other drug classes into the weight matrix. For the selected AEs, the top signals of single drug/drug combinations are listed in Table 4.7.

Note that if the spontaneous report mentioned the drug as "gadolinium" or "other contrast medium and gadolinium", instead of the exact generic drug names (GBCA 1, ..., GBCA 5), those reports are not treated as in the drug class in the illustration. The w_{ii^*} is 0 for the names like "gadolinium" or "other contrast medium and gadolinium". However, depending on the actual research interest, those names could be considered within the drug class and have different definitions of the weight matrix.

The gadolinium class including five GBCAs (not a single GBCA drug) is identified as the top signal for NSF and Fibrosis with very high relative reporting rates. Gadolinium (single drug signal) and Contrast medium and gadolinium (two drug collection signal) are ranked second and third signals for NSF, respectively. Single drug GBCA 5 (not the gadolinium class) with a RR of 29 is detected as the 2nd signal for Hypersensitivity. Moxifloxacin (single drug signal) is the top signal for Hypersensitivity (warning in the label for Moxifloxacin) with a RR of 20. Single drug GBCA 3 is the 7th signals detected for Hemodialysis with a RR of 10. The top signal for Hemodialysis (box warning in the label for Metformin) is Metformin (single drug signal) with a RR of 20.

"All Statins" as a class (not a single statin) is detected as a top signal (collection signal) for Myalgia, Rhabdomyolysis, increased Blood creatinine (CPK), and Muscular weakness, which is consistent with the information in the labels of the drugs. The relative reporting rates (of the Statins collection signal) are 15, 15, 13, 9 for Myalgia, Rhabdomyolysis, Blood creatinine increased, and Muscular weakness, respectively.

Ezetimbe (Ez) is found as signal (single drug signal) for Myalgia, Rhabdomyolysis, increased Blood CPK, muscular weakness in Table 4.7. In the label, Ez has adverse events including abnormal liver enzyme with elevated CPK level in blood, skeletal muscular effects (e.g., myopathy and rhabdomyolysis). The label also includes a warning that Ez should not be used with statins, which leads to muscle pain and weakness, and increased CPK.

Botulinum toxin type A has "generalized muscle weakness" in label, and RR of 19 in Table 4.7. Interferon Beta-1a has "muscle aches and tiredness" in the label and RR of 2 for muscular weakness. Gemfibrozil (Anon 2001) is known to have rhabdomyolysis and muscle pain/tenderness/weakness as side effects in some cases. From the FAERS data analysis, Gemfibrozil has RR of 46 for Rhabdomyolysis. Daptomycin (RR of 32 from FAERS data) is known to have musculoskeletal side effects: elevated creatine kinase (CK) levels, myalgia, muscle weakness. Ibandronic acid (RR of 7.7 from FAERS data) has known medical side effects including back pain, arm or leg pain, which are part of Myalgia. Fenofibrate (RR of 8.5 from FAERS data) has myopathy, Rhabdomyolysis, elevated CPK level, and renal failure in the label.

4.4 Notes and Discussion

- Different use of LRT method depending on different purpose

  Different types of applications using the LRT method are presented in this chapter. We show that the LRT method is highly flexible and that it can be used to detect signals in large and small data. Depending on the purpose of the safety study, one could conduct the LRT-based study using the FAERS data, or on a much smaller dataset including drugs within a drug class or AEs in an AE group.

- Interpretation and confirmation of the detected signals

  There are always a large number of drug-AE signals detected from the large safety databases. The signals could already be in label, or related with the indicated disease, or some treatment for the indicated disease. The signals could also appear due to the reporting system (error report, repeated cases, etc.), or off-label use. One drug-AE signal could be confounded with other signals. A lot of effort is needed to classify the identified signals. Sometimes, the researchers can restrict the analysis on a particular type of signal before the beginning of the exploration.

  It is also necessary to validate the identified signals by exploring the medical literature or regulatory documentation for possible support.

- LRT and Ext-LRT

  One of the advantages of the Ext-LRT is that the method can be used to find signals of multiple AEs (or drugs) with both the type-I error and false discovery rates controlled while retaining good power and sensitivity (the detailed simulation results are included in Ref. [149]). Note that in detecting signals among a drug class, the Ext-LRT tends to detect fewer signals than the basic LRT method (Chapter 3). The explanation is that, the threshold for the Ext-LRT is greater than or equal to those from each individual drug using the basic LRT, making Ext-LRT more conservative with fewer signals.

- Type-I error control for analysis over time

  In the work presented here, the overall type-I error control is not considered in evaluating the signals over time. However, when using the cumulative data (over time) repeatedly, it is necessary to control the overall type-I error using sequential methods, some of which are discussed in Chapter 6.

- Other definitions of weight matrix

  The weight matrix for the modified LRT can be defined according to the drug classes/AE groups as discussed in this chapter. It can also be constructed according to other factors of interest (e.g., dose, toxicity) or combinations of the factors. For example, the weight can be defined as 1 for drugs within a drug class and with similar doses, 0 for drugs within a drug class and with different level of doses. For some drugs (AEs) that do not belong to a drug class (or an AE group) of interest, but have similar toxicity (medically/biologically related), the weight can also be defined as 1. In this chapter, the weight is assigned values of 1 and 0 (related or not). It is also possible to explore different weight functions and values in order to reflect the degree of the relationship among the drugs and AEs, such as $\exp(-kd_{ii^*})$ or $\exp(-kd_{ii^*}^2)$, with d_{ii^*} denoting the distance between drugs i and i* based on their chemical structure or other factors of interest, and $k > 0$ a constant. The construction of the g-collections can consider the different weight information.

- Relationship between basic LRT, modified LRT, and Tree-based scan statistic (TBSS)

  As another method based on likelihood ratio test, a TBSS method [95], was used for drug safety data mining for data with hierarchical structure. The TBSS method Ref. [95] and the LRT method with different definitions of g (basic LRT and modified LRT methods) share similar features. All the three methods utilize likelihood ratio test with Poisson model and the null data are simulated using Multinomial distribution (Monte Carlo simulation) for p-value generation. Even though the modified LRT and the TBSS methods consider single AE (such as PT) and AE combinations, in the null data generation, the counts are generated for the single AE terms (such PTs) using multinomail distribution discussed in the basic LRT method (Chapter 3) and the counts for the AE combinations in the null data are the sum of the single AE counts.

  If the definition of the expected counts is the same, the Basic LRT method (discussed in Chapter 3 for AE signal detection for a fixed drug) is the same as the modified LRT with g as single AE term for a fixed drug and the TBSS method described in Ref. [95] (additional details in Appendix) for data with only one layer of the AE terms. The expected cell counts for LRT methods can be calculated using the fixed column total and the marginal row totals in the large $I \times J$ matrix from FAERS data or the exposure information associated with the observed adverse events if the exposure information is available (additional details on exposure information can be found in Chapter 6).

  Note that LRT methods can detect AE/AE collection signals for fixed drug of interest (as can TBSS), and can also detect drug/drug group signals for fixed AE of interest (which the TBSS cannot).

  Additional details about the TBSS method, and the relationship between the modified LRT method and the TBSS method are included in the Appendix.

4.5 Appendix: Tree-based Scan Statistic Method for AE Signals Evaluation

4.5.1 Summary of the method

The TBSS is a data mining method that simultaneously looks for excess risk in any of a large number of individual cells in a database as well as in groups of closely related cells, adjusting for the multiple testing inherent in the large number of overlapping groups evaluated [97]. It has previously been applied to occupational disease surveillance.

Kulldorff et al. [95] first applied this method to drug safety surveillance. According to [95], all diagnoses are first classified into a hierarchical tree structure. For each leaf i of the tree (finest granularity), the authors calculated the observed number c_i as well as the expected number n_i of AEs, adjusted for sex, age, and health plan. The total number of AEs $C = \sum_i c_i$ and the total expected count $N = \sum_i n_i$.

The next step involves making cuts on the branches of the tree. Each cut G defines a group of nearby and related leaves, and the sum of the observed and expected number of AEs on these leaves are denoted as c_G and n_G, respectively. Note that a single leaf is one potential cut. If $c_G/n_G > (C - c_G)/(N - n_G)$, there is a higher ratio of observed to expected AEs in the group defined by cut G compared with the rest of the tree. For each such cut G, the log likelihood ratio is calculated as

$$LLR(G) = c_G log(\frac{c_G}{n_G}) + (C - c_G)log(\frac{C - c_G}{N - n_G}).$$

The cut with the maximum log likelihood ratio is the most likely cluster of unexplained AEs, and its log likelihood ratio is the test statistic

$$T = max_G LLR(G).$$

4.5.2 Relationship to the LRT method

If we consider G as a single AE term (such as PT term). c_G is n_{ij^*}, and n_G is $E_{i.j^*}$ in basic LRT formulation for a fixed drug j^*. The T is the same as the $MLLR$ described in Section 3.1.2 (Chapter 3). For G as the g described in Section 4.3.1, the statistic from the tree-based scan method and the modified LRT should be same or similar depending on the way to obtain the expected counts.

Since the definition of the groups (such as AE collections) may be different, the detected signals may be different between the tree-based scan method and the LRT methods. In the modified LRT method, the AE collections are defined by the users through the weight matrix. The AE collections can be any combinations of the AE terms (such as PT term). One option is to define the g-collections according to MedDRA Structure (https://www.meddra.org/how-to-use/basics/hierarchy) for different layers such as System Organ Class (SOC), High Level Group Term (HLGT), or High Level Term (HLT). The names of the adverse events obtained from the safety data are usually Preferred Term (PT), which is the layer below HLT. If there are two layers of AEs in the data (for example PT and SOC), the modified LRT method may have AE collections as the single PT terms, or any combinations of PT terms if the PTs are within one SOC (including the SOC). The tree-based scan method also defines the tree leaves and branches using the MedDRA layers. In the data with only PT and SOC (two layers), the cuts may include all single PT terms and SOCs according to [95]. With the same layers and AE terms used in the modified LRT method and the TBSS method, the detected signals including single AE (such PT term) and AE collections should be consistent from the two methods. The group (G) defined by the TBSS method is actually one type of g-collections defined in the modified LRT method.

According to [95], statistical inference is conducted using Monte Carlo hypothesis testing [43], calculating the most likely cut in each random dataset. If the likelihood of the most likely cut in the real data is among the 5% highest of all the maximum values from the real and 99999 random datasets generated under the null hypothesis, then that cut constitutes a signal at the alpha = 0.05 statistical significance level. The Monte Carlo-based p-value is calculated as $p = R/(99999 + 1)$, where R is the rank of the log likelihood ratio from the most likely cut in the real dataset in relation to the log likelihood ratios from the most likely cuts in the random datasets.

In addition to the most likely cut, there are other cuts with more observed AEs than expected. To evaluate these statistically, they are compared with the most likely cut in the random datasets, to ensure that such secondary cuts can reject the null hypothesis on their own strength when they are statistically significant. This procedure is the same as the one used in LRT methods.

Wang et al. [138] extended the TBSS method to propensity score-matched tree-based scan statistic for evaluation of adverse drug events. This TBSS is similar to another LRT method for comparing AE issues between treatment and control groups described in Jung et al. [86]. Further details of the two methods are described in Chapter 8.

4.6 Tables and Figures

FIGURE 4.1
Weight matrix for drugs 1, 2, 3, and 4 and the definition of g as the collections of the drugs.

	1	2	3	4
1	1	1	0	1
2		1	0	1
3			1	0
4				1

Four drugs 1, 2, 3, 4.

1, 2, an 4 are in one drug class.

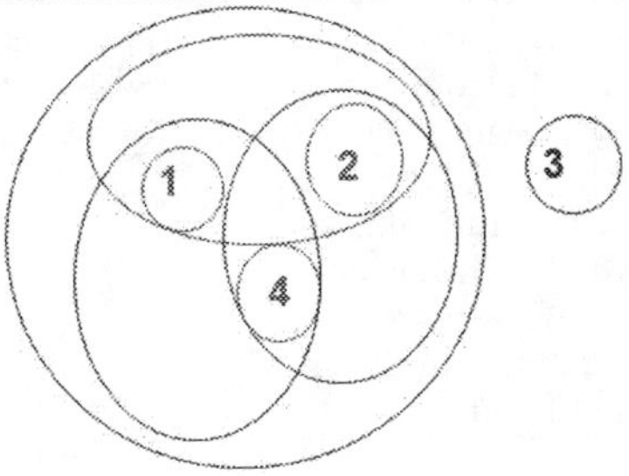

Each circle or ellipse represents one g.

TABLE 4.1
# of signals identified by different methods within the FAERS data and top signals detected by LRT method.

Year	Generic	#AE	PRR	sB.5	sB.01	sB.0001	BCPNN	LRT
0509	GBCA 1	998	296	102	130	141	154	91
0509	GBCA 2	326	131	45	71	74	62	40
0509	GBCA 3	719	242	62	118	127	104	58
0509	GBCA 4	482	188	38	82	94	60	36
0509	GBCA 5	430	145	53	84	87	79	49

AE signals detected by LRT for different drugs	
GBCA 1	NSF (RR=146), urticaria, sneezing, fibrosis, skin fibrosis, emotional dis, pruritus, scar, mobility decreased, skin3
GBCA 2	NSF (RR=294), emotional dis, fibrosis, scar, pain, mobility decreased, injury, skin fibrosis, anxiety, skin tightness, skin hypertrophy
GBCA 3	NSF (RR=826), fibrosis, emotional distress, skin fibrosis, scar, mobility decreased, pain, skin3
GBCA 4	NSF (RR=327), emotional distress, fibrosis, scar, pain, mobility decreased, skin fibrosis
GBCA 5	NSF (RR=147), hypersensitivity, vomiting, nausea, anaphylactoid, emotional distress, fibrosis, urticaria, scar, mobility decreased, skin fibrosis

#AE is the total number of AE (PT) names with at least one count for the listed drug. RR is estimated relative reporting rate. skin3 includes skin induration, skin hypertrophy, and skin tightness.

TABLE 4.2
# of signals identified by different methods within the drug class (suspect drug only).

Year	Genericn	#AE	PRR	sB.5	sB.01	BCPNN	LRT
05	GBCA 1	256	156	0	0	0	0
05	GBCA 2	70	30	0	1	0	0
05	GBCA 3	50	31	0	0	0	0
05	GBCA 4	28	27	1	5	1	1
05	GBCA 5	110	47	0	0	3	1
0507	GBCA 1	577	331	0	0	2	0
0507	GBCA 2	129	55	0	1	6	0
0507	GBCA 3	331	190	3	16	8	2
0507	GBCA 4	105	66	1	9	1	3
0507	GBCA 5	223	68	3	3	8	5
0509	GBCA 1	998	469	0	0	33	10
0509	GBCA 2	326	45	0	0	12	7
0509	GBCA 3	719	285	6	14	15	5
0509	GBCA 4	482	165	2	4	17	7
0509	GBCA 5	430	64	5	5	7	5

#AE is the total number of AE (PT) names with at least one count for the listed drug. Since sB.01 and sB.0001 have similar results, only sB.01 results are presented.

TABLE 4.3
Top signals for Gadolinium drugs and statins within the drug classes by LRT method.

GBCA 2	05	None (same for 0506 and 0507)
GBCA 2	0508	emotional distress (2.3), anxiety, injury, pain
GBCA 2	0509	pain (1.8), emotional distress, anxiety, injury, mobility decreased, scar
GBCA 3	05	None
GBCA 3	0506	NSF (RR=8.2)
GBCA 3	0507	NSF (RR=5.6), anixocytosis (6.4)
GBCA 3	0508	NSF (RR=3.7), hemodialysis (RR=4.9), dialysis (3.9), renal transplant (5.1), wheelchair use
GBCA 3	0509	NSF (RR=2.8), hemodialysis (RR=4.7), dialysis (4), renal transplant (4.6), wheelchair use
GBCA 4	05	post procedure complication (9.9)
GBCA 4	0506	ejection fraction decreased (RR=31), post procedure complication (9.9)
GBCA 4	0507	vertigo (35), ejection fraction decreased (RR=35), post procedure complication (9.8)
GBCA 4	0508	emotional distress (RR=3.0), injury, pain, anxiety, scar, fibrosis, mobility decreased
GBCA 4	0509	off label use (RR=5.8), pain, emotional distress (RR=1.5), anxiety, drug prescribing error, injury
GBCA 5	05	nausea (RR=2.8)
GBCA 5	0506	nausea (RR=2.9), hypersensitivity (RR=2.9), vomiting
GBCA 5	0507	nausea (2.6), hypersensitivity (RR=2.8), vomiting, urticaria, anaphylactoid reaction
GBCA 5	0508	hypersensitivity (RR=4.3), nausea (2.7), vomiting, anaphylactoid reaction, retching
GBCA 5	0509	hypersensitivity (RR=4.9), nausea, vomiting, anaphylactoid reaction, retching

RR is estimated relative reporting rate.

TABLE 4.4
Power, sensitivity and FDR for study of GBCA 5.

Measure	Year	η	PRR	BCPNN	sB.5	sB.01	LRT
Type-I error	2005	1	1	0.098	0.000	0.000	0.038
	2005–06	1	1	0.311	0.001	0.003	0.038
	2005–07	1	1	0.651	0.000	0.000	0.040
	2005–08	1	1	1.000	0.005	0.098	0.037
	2005–09	1	1	1.000	0.048	0.357	0.030
Power	2005	2	1	0.985	0.028	0.042	0.924
	2005–06	2	1	1.000	0.055	0.075	0.993
	2005–07	2	1	1.000	0.162	0.187	1.000
	2005–08	2	1	1.000	1.000	1.000	1.000
	2005–09	2	1	1.000	1.000	1.000	1.000
Power	2005	3	1	1.000	0.828	0.915	1.000
	2005–06	3	1	1.000	0.981	0.986	1.000
	2005–07	3	1	1.000	1.000	1.000	1.000
	2005–08	3	1	1.000	1.000	1.000	1.000
	2005–09	3	1	1.000	1.000	1.000	1.000
Sensitivity	2005	2	0.764	0.386	0.006	0.008	0.301
	2005–06	2	0.830	0.633	0.011	0.016	0.464
	2005–07	2	0.947	0.837	0.033	0.039	0.710
	2005–08	2	0.982	0.957	0.578	0.560	0.662
	2005–09	2	0.990	0.976	0.694	0.725	0.652
Sensitivity	2005	3	0.938	0.621	0.220	0.291	0.593
	2005–06	3	0.973	0.895	0.422	0.477	0.799
	2005–07	3	0.997	0.968	0.698	0.711	0.877
	2005–08	3	1.000	0.998	0.903	0.928	0.897
	2005–09	3	1.000	1.000	0.947	0.963	0.906
FDR	2005	2	0.937	0.008	0.000	0.000	0.004
	2005–06	2	0.947	0.027	0.000	0.000	0.002
	2005–07	2	0.961	0.005	0.000	0.000	0.000
	2005–08	2	0.962	0.120	0.001	0.007	0.000
	2005–09	2	0.964	0.227	0.004	0.033	0.000
FDR	2005	3	0.908	0.001	0.000	0.000	0.000
	2005–06	3	0.927	0.005	0.000	0.000	0.000
	2005–07	3	0.948	0.001	0.000	0.000	0.000
	2005–08	3	0.951	0.029	0.000	0.002	0.000
	2005–09	3	0.955	0.075	0.001	0.013	0.000

When η=1 FDR is type-I error and sensitivity is not defined.

TABLE 4.5
Number of signals detected by LRT-based methods and the percentage of true zeros.

Drug	LRT	Ext-LRT	Obs Zero
GBCA1	115	107	91.4
GBCA2	71	65	96.6
GBCA3	70	68	93.1
GBCA4	73	71	95.4
GBCA5	80	78	93.2

Obs Zero is the proportion of the observed zero in different drugs in GBCA class.

TABLE 4.6
Total common signals found by Ext-LRT for the five drugs in Gadolinium class in 2009–2013 dataset.

Drug	Common signals
GBCA1	NSF, skin induration, urticaria, skin hypertrophy, fibrosis, skin tightness, skin fibrosis, scar, mobility decrease, joint range of motion decrease, joint contracture, emotional distress, general physical health deterioration, pruritus
GBCA2	NSF, fibrosis, skin induration, skin hypertrophy, skin tightness, scar, skin fibrosis, mobility decreased, emotional distress, joint range of motion decreased, pain, general physical health deteriotation
GBCA3	NSF, fibrosis, skin induration, skin hypertrophy, skin fibrosis, skin tightness, scar, mobility decreased, emotional distress, joint range of motion decreased, joint contracture, general physical health deterioration, pain
GBCA4	NSF, fibrosis, skin hypertrophy, skin induration, skin tightness, skin fibrosis, scar, mobility decreased, emotional distress, joint range of motion decreased, joint contracture, general physical health deterioration, pain
GBCA5	NSF, fibrosis, skin hypertrophy, skin induration, skin tightness, skin fibrosis, scar, mobility decreased, joint contracture, joint range of motion decreased, emotional distress, pain, general physical health deterioration

TABLE 4.7
Signals of single drug or several drugs within drug classes by LRT method for selected AEs (a total of I=4273 drugs).

Selected AE	# drugs	# signals	top signal names
NSF	45	7	gadolinium class (RR=2739), Gadolinium (309), contrast medium and gadolinium (334), ...
Fibrosis	200	5	gadolinium class (RR=195), drug A (RR=36), Drug B (RR=18), ...
Hypersensitivity	1259	72	Moxifloxacin (RR=9), GBCA 5 (RR=29), Drug C (RR=8), Drug D (RR=5), Drug E (RR=14), ...
Hemodialysis	782	59	Metformin (RR=20), Drug F (RR=6), Drug G (RR=5), ..., GBCA 3 (RR=10, 7th order),...
Myalgia	1069	49	All Statins (15.5), Ezetimibe (16), Ezetimibe and simvastatin (15), Ibandronic acid (7.7), Drug I (4.8)
Rhabdomyolysis	907	60	All Statins (15.2), Ezetimibe (12.4), Ez and Simv (30), Fenofibrate (11.8), Gemfibrozil (46.1)
Blood creatine phosphokinase increased	947	66	All Statins (12.5), Daptomycin (32), Ez (14), Ez and Simvastatin (15), Fenofibrate (8.5)
Muscular weakness	1000	34	All Statins (8.7), Botulinum toxin type A (19), Ez (8), Ez and Sim (9), Interferon-beta-1a (2)

In the table, the # drugs are the drugs with non-zero count cells for the selected AEs. The computation is based on the data including all drugs (I) even though some AE-drug combinations have zero cell count. I is the same for all AEs in the drug-AE matrix. For signals not in the drugs label, drug A, B, C, etc. is used.

5

ZIP-LRT Method for Modeling Extra-zeros

A common feature of large safety databases in post-market surveillance is the large number of zero-cells in the data-matrix (drug-AE matrix). As discussed in Ref. [83], with more than 14,000 AEs (rows) and more than 6,000 drugs (columns), the percentage of drugs in the 2006–2011 FAERS database that have more than 90% of observed zero cells is as large as 88% (Figure 5.1 (left)).

The percentage of zero values ranges from 50.7% to 99.99%. For example, the two most commonly used blood thinners, namely Aspirin and Heparin, have the observed percentages of zero-cells as 54% and 75%, respectively; and Gadobenate Acid, a known contrast agent for magnetic resonance imaging (MRI), has observed percentage of zero-cells as 95%. It is important to take into account such high percentages of observed zero-cells in developing statistical signal detection methods. The ZIP-LRT model proposed by Huang et al. [83] for post-market data with a large number of zeros is discussed in this chapter.

5.1 ZIP-LRT Model

A Zero-Inflated Poisson Model can be used to model the true zeros that do not follow the Poisson distribution. Fix j, say the jth drug, and assume that the cell count, n_{ij}, corresponding to the ith AE, follows a Zero-Inflated Poisson(ZIP) model, $n_{ij} \sim ZIP(\omega_j, p_{ij})$; that is,

$$n_{ij} \sim \begin{cases} 0 & \text{with probability } \omega_j \\ Poisson(n_{i.}p_{ij}) & \text{with probability } (1 - \omega_j). \end{cases}$$

where $\omega_j (\geq 0)$ is the probability of observing a true zero, and it is assumed to depend on the jth drug.

For other AEs, as in the LRT, we continue to assume that

$$n_{.j} - n_{ij} \sim Poisson((n_{..} - n_{i.})q_{ij}).$$

Then, $P(n_{ij} = 0) = \omega_j + (1 - \omega_j)e^{-n_{i.}p_{ij}}$, and $P(n_{ij} = k) = \frac{e^{-n_{i.}p_{ij}}(n_{i.}p_{ij})^k(1-\omega_j)}{k!}$, when $k > 0$. We use Poisson model for $(n_{.j} - n_{ij})$ because the total counts for all other AEs, $(n_{.j} - n_{ij})$, is large. The parameter ω_j is assumed unknown and is treated as a nuisance parameter in the evaluation of AE signals associated with the jth drug. In what follows, since j is fixed, unless stated otherwise, we drop the index j in p_{ij}, q_{ij}, and ω_j, and consider the problem of testing H_0 vs. H_a, as above, but in the presence of the nuisance parameter, ω.

The likelihood function based on the ZIP model is

$$
\begin{aligned}
L(\omega, p_i, q_i) \quad &= \quad \prod_{i=1}^{I}[\{\omega + (1-\omega)e^{-n_{i.}p_i}\}^{u_i}\{(1-\omega)e^{-n_{i.}p_i}(n_{i.}p_i)^{n_{ij}}/n_{ij}!\}^{(1-u_i)} \\
&\times\{e^{-(n_{..}-n_{i.})q_i}[(n_{..}-n_{i.})q_i]^{(n_{.j}-n_{ij})}/(n_{.j}-n_{ij})!\}],
\end{aligned}
$$

where u_i=I$(n_{ij} = 0)$. Since, there are no closed forms for the MLEs of the parameters (ω, p_i, q_i), the Expectation-Maximization (EM) algorithm , as described in Lambert [100] and Hall [65], is used to obtain the MLEs under H_0 and H_a.

5.2 EM Algorithm for ZIP Model

First, we define unobservable latent random variables,

$$
z_i \sim \begin{cases} 1, & \text{when } n_{ij} \text{ is from a true zero.} \\ 0, & \text{when } n_{ij} \text{ is from } Poisson(n_{i.}p_i). \end{cases}
$$

Next, under H_0 and H_a separately, we apply the EM algorithm [141] as follows to find the MLEs of the parameters (ω, p_i, q_i).

- Under H_0:

  Let z_i be labeled as z_{i0}, $i = 1, ..., I$. If we could observe $\underline{z} = (z_{10}, \cdots, z_{I0})$, the complete log-likelihood function can be written as

$$
\begin{aligned}
&log(L_0) = l_c(\underline{z}, \omega, p_0) \\
&\propto \sum_{i=1}^{I}[z_{i0}\text{log}(\omega) + (1-z_{i0})\text{log}(1-\omega) + (1-z_{i0})(-n_{i.}p_0 + n_{ij}\text{log}p_0)] \\
&+\sum_{i=1}^{I}[-(n_{..}-n_{i.})p_0 + (n_{.j}-n_{ij})\text{log}p_0] \\
&= l_c(\underline{z}, \omega) + l_c(\underline{z}, p_0)
\end{aligned}
$$

  Note that the complete log-likelihood, $l_c(\underline{z}, \omega, p_0)$, factors as sum of two terms, one containing $(\underline{z}, \omega)$; and the other containing $(\underline{z}, p_0)$. EM algorithm can be used to maximize $l_c(\underline{z}, \omega, p_0)$ by alternating between the expectation step (E-step), in which $\underline{z}$ is estimated by its expectation under the current estimates of p_0 and ω, and the maximization step (M-step), in which $l_c(\underset{\sim}{z}, \omega, p_0)$ is evaluated at the current estimate of $\underset{\sim}{z}$ maximized with respect to p_0 and ω.

E-step Estimate z_{i0} by its conditional expectation, at the (r+1)th iteration:

$$\begin{aligned}
\hat{z_{i0}}^{(r+1)} &= E(z_{i0} = 1|n_{ij}) \\
&= \text{P}(\text{zero state}|n_{ij}, \hat{p_0}^{(r)}, \hat{\omega}^{(r)}) \\
&= \frac{\text{P}(n_{ij}|\text{zero state})\text{P}(\text{zero state})}{\text{P}(n_{ij}|\text{zero state})\text{P}(\text{zero state}) + \text{P}(n_{ij}|Poisson, \hat{p_0}^{(r)})\text{P}(Poisson, \hat{p_0}^{(r)})} \\
&= \begin{cases} \frac{\hat{\omega}^{(r)}}{\hat{\omega}^{(r)} + e^{-n_{i.}\hat{p_0}^{(r)}}(1-\hat{\omega}^{(r)})}, & \text{if } n_{ij} = 0 \\ 0, & \text{if } n_{ij} > 0 \end{cases}
\end{aligned}$$

M-step i) The estimate of ω, for given $\hat{\underset{\sim}{z}}^{(r+1)} = (z_{10}^{(r+1)}, \cdots, z_{I0}^{(r+1)})$ at the (r+1)th iteration, is

$$\hat{\omega}^{(r+1)} = \frac{\sum_{i=1}^{I} \hat{z_{i0}}^{(r+1)}}{I}.$$

ii) The estimate of p_0, for given $\hat{\underset{\sim}{z}}^{(r+1)}$ at the (r+1)th iteration, is

$$\hat{p_0}^{(r+1)} = \frac{\sum_{i=1}^{I}[(1 - \hat{z_{i0}}^{(r+1)})n_{ij} + (n_{,j} - n_{ij})]}{\sum_{i=1}^{I}[(1 - \hat{z_{i0}}^{(r+1)})n_{i.} + (n_{..} - n_{i.})]}.$$

Let $(\hat{\omega}, \hat{z}_{i0}, \hat{p}_0)$ denote the MLEs of (ω, z_{i0}, p_0), under H_0, obtained using the above EM algorithm.

- Under H_a:

  The complete log-likelihood function is,

$$\begin{aligned}
\log(\text{L}_a) &\propto \sum_{i=1}^{I}[z_i\log(\omega) + (1 - z_i)\log(1 - \omega) + (1 - z_i)(-n_{i.}p_i + n_{ij}\log p_i)] \\
&\quad + \sum_{i=1}^{I}[-(n_{..} - n_{i.})q_i + (n_{.j} - n_{ij})\log q_i] \\
&= l_c(\underset{\sim}{z}, \omega) + l_c(\underset{\sim}{z}, \underset{\sim}{p}) + l_c(\underset{\sim}{q}),
\end{aligned}$$

with $\underset{\sim}{p} = (p_1, \cdots, p_I)$ and $\underset{\sim}{q} = (q_1, \cdots, q_I)$. Thus log (L_a) factors as the sum of three terms. The first term contains $(\underset{\sim}{z}, \omega)$; and the second term contains $(\underset{\sim}{z}, \underset{\sim}{p})$; the third term contains $\underset{\sim}{q}$. The EM algorithm can be used to find the MLEs, as follows:

E-step Estimate z_i by its conditional expectation, at the (r+1)th iteration. This is the same as that given under H_0:

$$\tilde{z_i}^{(r+1)} = E(z_i = 1|n_{ij}) = \begin{cases} \frac{\tilde{\omega}^{(r)}}{\tilde{\omega}^{(r)} + e^{-n_{i.}\tilde{p_i}^{(r)}}(1-\tilde{\omega}^{(r)})}, & \text{if } n_{ij} = 0 \\ 0, & \text{if } n_{ij} > 0. \end{cases}$$

M-step

i) Estimate $\tilde{\omega}^{(r+1)}$ of ω, obtained by maximizing $l_c(\tilde{\underline{z}}^{(r+1)}, \omega)$, for given $\tilde{\underline{z}}^{(r+1)}$ at the (r+1)th iteration, is

$$\tilde{\omega}^{(r+1)} = \frac{\sum_{i=1}^{I} \tilde{z_i}^{(r+1)}}{I}.$$

ii) Estimate $\tilde{p_i}^{(r+1)}$ of p_i, obtained by maximizing $l_c(\tilde{z_i}^{(r+1)}, p_i)$, for given $\tilde{\underline{z}}^{(r+1)}$ at the (r+1)th iteration, is

$$\frac{\mathrm{d}l_c(\tilde{z_i}^{(r+1)}, p_i)}{\mathrm{d}p_i} = (1 - \tilde{z_i}^{(r+1)})(-n_{i.} + n_{ij}/p_i),$$

giving,

$$\tilde{p_i}^{(r+1)} = n_{ij}/n_{i.}\ , \text{ since } (1 - \tilde{z_i}^{(r+1)}) > 0.$$

iii) Estimate $\tilde{q_i}^{(r+1)}$ of q_i, obtained by maximizing $l_c(q_i)$ at the (r+1)th iteration, is

$$\frac{\mathrm{d}l_c(q_i)}{\mathrm{d}q_i} = -(n_{..} - n_{i.}) + (n_{.j} - n_{ij})/q_i,$$

giving

$$\tilde{q_i}^{(r+1)} = (n_{.j} - n_{ij})/(n_{..} - n_{i.}).$$

Note that the MLEs of p_i and q_i under H$_a$, are the same as their MLEs obtained from the basic LRT method. Also,

$$\tilde{z_i}^{(r+1)} = \begin{cases} \frac{\tilde{\omega}^{(r)}}{\tilde{\omega}^{(r)} + e^{-n_{ij}}(1-\tilde{\omega}^{(r)})}, & \text{if } n_{ij} = 0 \\ 0, & \text{if } n_{ij} > 0. \end{cases}$$

Since

$$\tilde{\omega}^{(r+1)} = \frac{\sum_{i=1}^{I} \tilde{z_i}^{(r+1)}}{I} \leq \tilde{\omega}^{(r)},$$

the iteration converges when $\tilde{\omega} = 0$. Thus, we have the following lemma.

Lemma 5.2.1 *Under H_a, the maximum likelihood estimates of p_i and q_i converge to the values obtained from the LRT method.*

It follows from the lemma that the likelihood function under H$_a$ is maximized when $\tilde{z_i} = 0$ and that the maximum likelihood estimate of ω is $\tilde{\omega} = 0$.

5.3 Likelihood Ratio Test Statistic

The likelihood ratio, for ith AE and the fixed jth drug, is

$$\begin{aligned}\widetilde{LR}_{ij} &= \frac{\mathrm{L}_a(\tilde{p}_i, \tilde{q}_i)}{\mathrm{L}_0(\hat{\omega}, \hat{z_{i0}}, \hat{p_0})} \\ &= [\hat{\omega}^{\hat{z_{i0}}}(1-\hat{\omega})^{(1-\hat{z_{i0}})}]^{(-1)}[e^{-n_{i.}\hat{p_0}}(n_{i.}\hat{p_0})^{n_{ij}}/n_{ij}!]^{\hat{z_{i0}}} \\ &\times e^{(n_{..}\hat{p_0}-n_{.j})}(\frac{n_{ij}}{n_{i.}})^{n_{ij}}(\frac{n_{.j}-n_{ij}}{n_{..}-n_{i.}})^{(n_{.j}-n_{ij})}/(\hat{p_0}^{n_{.j}}), i=1,\cdots,I.\end{aligned} \tag{1}$$

The likelihood ratio test statistic for H_0 vs. H_a is $\widetilde{\mathrm{MLLR}} = \max_i(\widetilde{logLR_{ij}}I(\tilde{p}_{ij} > \tilde{q}_{ij}))$. The relationship between LRT method and ZIP LRT method is as follows:

If $n_{ij} = 0$ and $\hat{z_{i0}} \neq 0$, $\tilde{p}_i < \tilde{q}_i$. In this case, we let $\log\widetilde{LR}_{ij} = logLR_{ij} = 0$, as we are only interested in $\tilde{p}_i > \tilde{q}_i$.

If $n_{ij} > 0$, then $\hat{z_{i0}} = 0$, and

$$\begin{aligned}\widetilde{\mathrm{LR}}_{ij} &= (1-\hat{\omega})^{(-1)}e^{n_{..}\hat{p_0}-n_{.j}}[(\frac{\tilde{p}_i}{\hat{p_0}})^{n_{ij}}(\frac{\tilde{q}_i}{\hat{p_0}})^{(n_{.j}-n_{ij})}] \\ &= (1-\hat{\omega})^{(-1)}e^{(n_{..}\hat{p_0}-n_{.j})}[(\frac{n_{.j}}{n_{..}})/\hat{p_0}]^{n_{.j}} \\ &\quad [(\frac{n_{ij}}{n_{i.}})^{n_{ij}}(\frac{n_{.j}-n_{ij}}{n_{..}-n_{i.}})^{(n_{.j}-n_{ij})}/(\frac{n_{.j}}{n_{..}})^{n_{.j}}] \\ &= (1-\hat{\omega})^{(-1)}e^{(n_{..}\hat{p_0}-n_{.j})}[(\frac{n_{.j}}{n_{..}})/\hat{p_0}]^{n_{.j}}\mathrm{LR}_{ij},\end{aligned}$$

where $LR_{ij*} = LR_{ij}$ defined in Chapter 3 (Equations 3.1 and 3.2). Therefore, we have

Lemma 5.3.1 *If* $n_{ij} > 0$,

$$log\widetilde{LR}_{ij} - logLR_{ij} = -log(1-\hat{\omega}) + n_{..}\hat{p_0} - n_{.j} + n_{.j}log[(\tfrac{n_{.j}}{n_{..}})/\hat{p_0}] \geq 0.$$

5.4 Stratified ZIP LRT

To incorporate the effect of binary or categorical factors such as age groups and gender, first define,

$$\begin{aligned}U_0 &= \frac{\sum_{i=1}^{I}[(1-\hat{z_{i0}})n_{ij} + (n_{.j}-n_{ij})]}{\sum_{i=1}^{I}[(1-\hat{z_{i0}})E_{ij} + (n_{.j}-E_{ij})]} \\ &= n_{.j}/[n_{.j} - (\sum_{i=1}^{I}\hat{z}_{i0}E_{ij})/I].\end{aligned}$$

Then, the likelihood ratio of ith AE and jth drug can be rewritten as

$$\widetilde{\mathrm{LR}}_{ij} = [\hat{\omega}^{\hat{z_{i0}}}(1-\hat{\omega})^{(1-\hat{z_{i0}})}]^{(-1)}[e^{-E_{ij}U_0}(E_{ij}U_0)^{n_{ij}}/n_{ij}!]^{\hat{z_{i0}}}$$
$$[\frac{e^{-n_{.j}(1-U_0)}}{{U_0}^{n_{.j}}}](\frac{n_{ij}}{E_{ij}})^{n_{ij}}[\frac{n_{.j}-n_{ij}}{n_{.j}-E_{ij}}]^{(n_{.j}-n_{ij})}$$

Now, from Lemma 5.3.1, if $n_{ij} > 0$, then $\hat{z_{i0}} = 0$, and

$$\log(\widetilde{\mathrm{LR}}_{ij}) = -\log(1-\hat{\omega}) + \log[\frac{e^{-n_{.j}(1-U_0)}}{{U_0}^{n_{.j}}}] + \log(\frac{n_{ij}}{E_{ij}})^{n_{ij}} + \log[\frac{n_{.j}-n_{ij}}{n_{.j}-E_{ij}}]^{(n_{.j}-n_{ij})}.$$

Let M be the total number of strata formed by the covariates (gender, age groups, etc.) under consideration. Let $log\widetilde{\mathrm{LR}}_{ij}^{(m)}$ be the value of $log\widetilde{\mathrm{LR}}_{ij}$ for stratum m ($m = 1, \cdots, M$) obtained by replacing E_{ij} and ω by $E_{ij}^{(m)}$ and $\omega^{(m)}$, respectively, where $E_{ij}^{(m)} = n_{i.}^{(m)} n_{.j}^{(m)} / n_{..}^{(m)}$ and $\omega^{(m)}$ is the MLE of ω.

Then, $log\widetilde{\mathrm{LR}}_{ij}^{(M)}$ is defined as the weighted average of $log(\widetilde{LR}_{ij}^{(m)}), m = 1, \cdots, M$, with weights being proportional to the total number of reports, $n_{..}^{(m)}$, in the stratum m, where $\widetilde{LR}_{ij}^{(m)}$ denotes $\widetilde{LR}_{ij}$ computed from the stratum m: That is,

$$log(\widetilde{LR}_{ij}^{(M)}) = \sum_{m=1}^{M} \frac{n_{..}^{(m)}}{n_{..}} log(\widetilde{LR}_{ij}^{(m)}).$$

The test statistic is then $\widetilde{MLLR} = max_i(log(\widetilde{LR}_{ij}^{(M)}))$. Note that $max_i(logLR_{ij}^{(m)})$ can be used to detect signals from stratum m. This method is used in Section 5.7.

5.5 Hypothesis Testing

To carry out the hypothesis test, we use Monte Carlo simulation to find the distribution of $\widetilde{MLLR}$ under H_0 in the presence of the nuisance parameter ω. In order to simulate the data under H_0, first we estimate the probability of true zeros (ω) for the jth drug using the ZIP model, and then use Bernoulli process:

$$z_{i0} \sim^{iid} Bernoulli(\hat{\omega}I/I_0), i = 1, \cdots, I_0(\leq I).$$

Here, $\hat{\omega}I/(I_0)$ denotes the estimate of the conditional probability of true zeros given an observed zero (i.e., relative proportion of true zero cells among the observed zero cells), I_0 is the total number of cells with observed zeros for the jth drug, and I is the total number of AEs. If $\sum_{i=1}^{I_0} z_{i0} = k$, there are k true zeros, at the indexes $(i_1, i_2, \cdots i_k)$, according to the above Bernoulli process, where we assign $n_{i_1 j} = n_{i_2 j} = \cdots = n_{i_k j} = 0$.

The number of counts for each AE among the cells not assigned as true zero cells is then simulated using a Multinomial distribution assigning relative reporting rate as 1 for all the cells excluding the true zero cells. Let us label the remaining (non-true zero) cells as $i = 1, \cdots, I_k$, where $I_k = I - k$. Then the joint distribution of cell counts $(n_{1j}, \cdots, n_{I_k,j})$, conditional on $n_{.j}$ and I_k, is

$$(n_{1j}, \cdots, n_{I_k,j})|n_{.j,I_k} \sim Multinomial(n_{.j}, (\frac{n_{1.}}{n_{I_k}}, \cdots, \frac{n_i}{n_{I_k}}, \cdots, \frac{n_{I_k.}}{n_{I_k}})), \quad (5.2)$$

where n_{I_k} is the sum of marginal row totals that do not include the true zero cells.

A total the of 9,999 Multinomial datasets under H_0 are simulated using the process described in the above Equation, and 10,000 $\widetilde{MLLR}$s are calculated (9,999 values calculated from the simulated datasets and one from the observed dataset). If the value of $\widetilde{MlLR}$ from the observed dataset is greater than the 95th percentile of the 10,000 $\widetilde{MLLR}$ values (objective threshold), the null hypothesis is rejected at the $\alpha = 0.05$ level. The corresponding p-value is calculated as 1-R/(1+9999), where R is the rank of the $\widetilde{MlLR}$ value for the observed dataset among all 10,000 $\widetilde{MLLR}$ values.

If the p-value of $\widetilde{MLLR}$ is less than one-sided level of significance, $\alpha = 0.05$ for the FAERS dataset, the AEs associated with $\widetilde{MLLR} = \max_i \widetilde{logLR}_{ij}$ (i.e., the largest $\widetilde{logLR}_{ij}$) are the (strongest) signals for the jth drug under consideration. Once we reject the null hypothesis (H_0 based on the largest $\widetilde{logLR}_{ij}$), the type-I error α is saved and allows us to apply that saved α to identify other signals by moving to the second largest $\widetilde{logLR}_{ij}$, the third largest $\widetilde{logLR}_{ij}$, and so on. The AEs corresponding to the second largest $\widetilde{logLR}_{ij}$ value, the third largest $\widetilde{logLR}_{ij}$ value, and so on, could be declared as signals if their p-values are less than 0.05. Note that the detection of these additional signals only impacts the false discovery rate (FDR), not the type-I error. Also, note that we are not implying the control of type-I error in the context of multiple testing as there are no multiple null and alternative hypotheses being tested here. Theorem 5.5.1 below, whose proof is deferred to the Appendix, shows that the FDR is always less than or equal to the type-I error.

Theorem 5.5.1 *ZIP LRT method asymptotically controls both the type-I error and false discovery rates.*

5.6 Simulation Study

In this section, we evaluate the finite sample size performance of the ZIP LRT method for signal detection using several characteristics namely, the power, type-I error rate, sensitivity, and false discovery rate (FDR) (definitions are presented in Section 3.2.2).

5.6.1 Data simulation

We simulate datasets with/without signals, and with/without some pre-specified true zeros, using the marginal counts from the 2006–2011 FAERS database (details of the data are provided in Section 5.7). We simulate data with 14,415 rows, and the same marginal totals ($n_{i.}$) from the 2006–2011 data, using the steps below.

First, the percentage of the true zero cells is assumed to be given (ω), and true zeros ($z_i = 1$) are simulated using Bernoulli process as follows:

$$z_i \sim^{iid} Bernoulli(\omega) \; i = 1, \cdots, I.$$

If $z_i = 1$, assign $n_{ij} = 0$ (true zero for ith AE). For the rest of cells with $z_i = 0$, under the null hypothesis the data are simulated using (Equation 5.2), and under the alternative hypothesis (higher relative reporting rate for 5 pre-specified AEs), the data are simulated using the following:

$$(n_{1j}, \cdots, n_{Lj})|n_{.j} \sim Multinomial(n_{.j}, (\eta_1 \times r_0 \times \frac{n_{1.}}{n_L}, \cdots, \eta_L \times r_0 \times \frac{n_{L.}}{n_L}), \tag{5.3}$$

where $n_L = \sum_{i'=1}^{L} n_{i'.}$, with L as the number of cells not identified as true zero cells. The constraint is that $0 \leq \eta_i \times r_0 \times \frac{n_{i.}}{n_L} \leq 1$, and $\sum_{i=1}^{L} \eta_i \times r_0 \times \frac{n_{i.}}{n_L} = 1$. Here, r_0 is interpreted as the baseline risk, which may vary with different datasets. The selected AEs, designated as true signals, are assigned values of η higher than 1, and the other non-selected AEs (among non-true zero cells) are assigned values of η equal to 1. Details on the relationship between η and relative reporting rates are provided in Section 3.2.1.

We evaluate how the percentage of true zeros, the η among the non-true zero cells, the sample size ($n_{.j}$), and the number of true signals affect the performance of the ZIP LRT method. The percentage of true zeros (ω) for a drug is assigned to be 0%, 30%, 50%, or 70%. We notice that a single true signal leads to a slightly higher sensitivity compared with multiple true signals and that the sensitivity also depends on other factors, such as the marginal row totals ($n_{i.}$) and the sample size ($n_{.j}$). Here, we only present results for five AEs as true signals. The marginal row totals ($n_{i.}$) of the five AEs are taken to be 49425, 51307, 59289, 62618, and 77154, respectively, which fall within the

75th - 85th percentile range of the marginal totals from the 2006-2011 FAERS data. Under the null hypothesis, all the AEs (excluding the ones with the true zeros) are assigned $\eta = 1$. Under the alternative hypothesis, the five signals are assigned the same value of η (equal to $3, 3.5, 4, 4.5$, or 6), and the other AEs, excluding the AEs with the true zero cells, are assigned η equal to 1.

The sample sizes ($n_{.j}$) are taken to be 600, 1000, 3000, 6000, and 12000 to represent drugs with varying sample sizes.

5.6.2 Simulation results

The simulation results (with 1000 repeats) including power, sensitivity, and FDR for different scenarios are presented in Tables 5.1 to 5.3. When all n_{ij} are generated from Poisson distribution (with $\omega = 0$) (Table 5.1), $\hat{\omega}$ from the ZIP LRT is close to 0, and both the ZIP LRT and LRT methods have similar performance characteristics. The type-I error (power when $\eta = 1$) is 0.036 for the ZIP LRT and is 0.038 for the LRT method. The power is 100% for both the methods when there are five true signals with the relative reporting rate, $\eta = 4$.

As shown in Table 5.2, when the values of ω vary from 0% to 90%, with large sample size of 12,000 and the η values, for the five true signals as 4, the ZIP LRT method shows 100% power, high sensitivity (≥ 0.9) and low FDR (< 0.05). The sensitivity becomes slightly lower for cases with higher ω (50% - 90%). A similar pattern is observed for moderate sample size of 6,000.

When sample size is moderate (6,000) and the value of ω is 50%, both the power and sensitivity increase, while FDR decreases, with increasing values of the sample size and the η values (Table 5.3). When the value of η is 1, i.e., there are no signals in the data, both the type-I error and FDR are less than the pre-specified $\alpha = 0.05$ level.

5.7 Application to 2006-2011 FAERS Data

5.7.1 Estimated percentage of true zeros

The probability of true zero cells ($\hat{\omega}$), by drug, is obtained by applying the proposed ZIP model for the 2006–2011 FAERS data with all drugs and AEs. A total of 6,928 drugs were evaluated. The estimated percentage of true zero cells was much smaller than the observed percentage of zero cells, by drug, as shown in Figure 5.1 (with a high frequency for observed zero percentages between 90–100% in Figure 5.1 (left), versus a high frequency of estimated true zero percentages from the ZIP model between 10–40% in Figure 5.1 (right)). This discrepancy is expected as for a large number of drugs, the observed zeros may contain only a few true zeros.

5.7.2 Application to selected drugs

The ZIP LRT and LRT methods were applied to the 2006–2011 FAERS data with suspect and concomitant drugs in order to detect AE signals with higher reporting ratios. We selected six drugs, with varying sample sizes ($n_{.j}$) and percentages of observed zeros (Table 5.4). Prednisone is used for treating inflammatory disease and some types of cancer, with AEs including increased blood sugar for diabetics, immunosuppression, depression, osteonecrosis, facial swelling, etc. Aspirin is used for reducing the risk of stroke in patients, with AEs including bleeding, nausea, headache, dyspepsia, diarrhea, etc. Heparin acts as an anticoagulant, preventing the formation of clots and extension of existing clots within the blood, with AEs including Hemorrhage, Hypersensitivity, Thrombocytopenia, Thrombosis, etc. Prednisone, Aspirin, and Heparin have been approved by the FDA in the mid-1900s, and have large sample sizes ($n_{.j}$) in the FAERS database. Gadopentetic acid (first approval in 1988) is used for Magnetic Resonance Imaging (MRI) of the brain, spine, and body, with AEs including Nephrogenic systemic fibrosis (NSF), hypersensitivity, renal failure, nausea, headache, etc. Gadobenate acid (first approval in 2004) is for MRI of the brain and spine, with AEs including NSF, hypersensitivity, nausea, headache, etc. Docosanol (first approval in 2000) is for treating cold sore, with AEs including skin irritation, headache, acne, burning, itching, swelling, dryness, etc.

Table 5.4 gives the number of signals detected by the ZIP LRT and the LRT methods, percentages of observed zeros, and the estimates of the percentages of true zeros. When the estimated $\hat{\omega}$ is small, the number of signals from the ZIP LRT method is similar to that from the LRT method. As $\hat{\omega}$ increases, the difference between the number of signals detected by the LRT and the ZIP LRT methods also increases. When $\hat{\omega}$ is large, the ZIP LRT method leads to a smaller number of signals compared to those with the LRT method, as a result of adjustment for the percent of true zeros (nuisance parameter). Table 5.5 gives the signals for the drug Gadobenate detected by both the ZIP LRT and LRT up to the last significant AE signal detected by the ZIP LRT. The order of AE signals by the two methods is the same. Additional 43 signals detected by the LRT method are not shown in the table (Table 5.5). The p-values of AE signals associated with the LRT method are all < 0.0001 whereas the ones associated with the ZIP LRT method are < 0.0001 up to "Extremity contracture", and for the last four AE signals the p-values are 0.0003, 0.0037, 0.0069, and 0.0210, respectively.

The results of ZIP LRT stratified analysis with gender (F: Female, M:Male, U:Unknown) conducted for two drugs namely Gadobenate acid and Docosnol are presented in Table 5.6. Without stratification the number of signals detected by the ZIP LRT method for Gadobenate acid and Docosanol were 27 and 8, respectively. More signals were detected for the two drugs (29 for Gadobenate acid and 15 for Docosanol respectively) with the ZIP LRT stratified analysis. For Gadobenate acid, the number of AE signals for female was

28 and that for male was 26. Four of the 28 signals detected for female were not detected in male, and 2 of the 26 signals detected for male were not detected in female. The rest of the 24 signals were common for male and female, although their order was not the same. While there was no significant effect of gender on the number of signals detected for Gadobenate acid, it may have a significant effect for Docosanol since the number of signals detected for female was 20 and that for male was 5. Also, the 5 signals detected for male were the first five signals for female.

The ZIP LRT results presented in Tables 5.4 to 5.6 are exploratory in nature, and a causal inference on signals detected can be established only after a careful clinical investigation of the individual reports validated through other datasets. A thorough investigation of a signal detected by statistical methods such as the LRT or the ZIP LRT can lead to changes in the drug label.

5.8 Notes and Discussion

The ZIP LRT method for signal detection is developed for the drugs from the FAERS database with a large number of zero cell-counts. For large sample sizes, the ZIP LRT is shown to control both the type-I error and FDR, with adjustment of the possible true zeros. Simulation study was used to evaluate the performance of the ZIP LRT with varying percentages of true zeros, sample sizes, and relative reporting rates.

The ZIP LRT method is recommended instead of the LRT method for, a high percentage of observed zeros in the data and a large estimate of ω, since the ZIP LRT method gives fewer number of signals than the LRT method, and the order of signals from the two methods remains the same. When the estimates of ω is close to 0, the ZIP LRT method gives results similar to the LRT. This can also be seen theoretically, since when $\omega = 0$, n_{ij} in ZIP model follows Poisson model, and the ZIP LRT and the LRT test statistics become identical. That is, when $\omega = 0$, $z_{i0} = 0$, $\hat{p}_0 = n_{.j}/n_{..}$, and $\widetilde{logLR_{ij}}(ZIP) - logLR_{ij}(LRT) = 0$.

The proposed method was also applied to other drugs with small sample sizes, such as Cortisone (with $n_{.j} = 45$) and Amoxapin (with $n_{.j} = 58$), where most of the nonzero observed cell-counts are 1 's and the percentage of observed zeros is very large ($> 99\%$) (results not shown). The estimates of ω for these drugs are very small ($< 6\%$). When the observed percentage of zeros is large and the remaining cell counts are small such as 1's and 2's (such as for a newly approved drug), the EM algorithm may take long time to converge and may be computationally challenging.

Note that the ZIP-LRT test statistic discussed in this chapter is $\widetilde{MLLR} = \max_i \widetilde{logLR_{ij}}$ for a fixed $j = j^*$. The MLLR is obtained by maximizing the

$\widetilde{logLR}_{ij}$ over $i = 1, \cdots, I$. The null data for statistical inference is generated for one column ($j = j^*$). For signal detection among drug classes, Zhao et al. [149] extended the ZIP-LRT to Ext-ZIP-LRT by obtaining the statistic as $MMLLR = max_j(MLR_j) = max_j(max_i(LR_{ij}))$, where maximum is taken over $i = 1, \ldots I$ and $j = 1, \cdots, J$. The null data simulated will follow the same approach for the ZIP-LRT, but will be simulated for all columns ($j = 1, \cdots, J$). The Ext-ZIP-LRT detects signals of drug-AE combinations in the whole data including drugs within one drug class (instead of AE signals in one fixed drug). From Ref. [149], Ext-ZIP-LRT is more conservative than ZIP-LRT due to the higher threshold value (obtained from the whole data).

Finally, the derivation of ZIP-LRT type test statistics for testing H_0 vs. H_a can be carried out for other zero-inflated models using the EM algorithm. For example, to incorporate the dependence and the heterogeneity among the n_{ij}'s, let $n_{ij}|\theta, \omega \sim ZIP(\omega, p_{ij}\theta), (n_{.j} - n_{ij})|\theta \sim Poisson((n_{..} - n_{i.})q_{ij}\theta)$, where $\theta \sim Gamma(\beta, \beta)$, with mean 1 and variance $1/\beta$, so that for $0 \leq \beta \leq 1$ the variance of θ is large. This formulation leads to a Zero-inflated Negative Binomial (ZINB) model for n_{ij}. If the parameter β is known and $\beta = 1$, say, the LRT test for ZINB is same as that for ZIP model. If β is unknown, the EM algorithm is to be implemented on all the unknown parameters including the nuisance parameters ω and β.

One can construct ZIP model for Bayesian methods. The ZIP model includes a proportion p_0 of true-zeros and a proportion $(1 - p_0) \times (e^{-\lambda_{ij}E_{ij}})$ of zeros coming from the Poisson distribution , $Poisson(\lambda_{ij}E_{ij})$. That is

$$n_{ij} = \begin{cases} 0 & \text{with probability } p_0 \\ Poisson(\lambda_{ij}E_{ij}) & \text{with probability } (1 - p_0) \end{cases}$$

In the Bayesian approach (of ZIP-DP method), the probability p_0 can be assigned a fixed value or a Beta prior, and λ_{ij}, as DP prior for ZIP-DP method and as single gamma prior for ZIP-sB method.

5.9 Appendix: Proof of Theorem 5.5.1

First assume the case where p_0 and w are known. As mentioned in Lemma 5.3.1, the relationship between log$\widetilde{LR}_{ij}$ and logLR_{ij}, corresponding to ZIP LRT and LRT methods, is given by,

log$\widetilde{LR}_{ij}$-logLR_{ij}=-log$(1-\omega)+n_{..}p_0-n_{.j}+n_{.j}log[(\frac{n_{.j}}{n_{..}})/p_0]\geq 0$.

Define, $f=$ -log$(1-\omega)+n_{..}p_0-n_{.j}+n_{.j}log[(\frac{n_{.j}}{n_{..}})/p_0]$. Then $f\geq 0$, and $\max_{1\leq i\leq I}$(logLR_{ij})=$\max_{1\leq i\leq I}$(log$\widetilde{LR}_{ij}$)-$f(\omega,p_0)$.

Also, let T be the threshold from the empirical null distribution for $\max_i$(logLR$_{ij}$). Since the LRT method controls the type-I error,

$$\mathrm{P}(\ \max_i(\mathrm{logLR}_{ij})>\mathrm{T}|\mathrm{H}_0)\leq\alpha.$$

Let $\widetilde{T}$ be the threshold from the empirical null distribution, adjusted for the nuisance parameter ω; that is, let $\widetilde{T}=T+f(\omega,p_0)$. Then, we have

$$\begin{aligned} & P(\max_i(log\widetilde{LR}_{ij}))>\widetilde{T}|H_0) \\ = \ & P(\max_i(log\widetilde{LR}_{ij})-f(\omega,p_0)>\widetilde{T}-f(\omega,p_0)|H_0) \\ = \ & P(\max_i(logLR_{ij}))>T|H_0)\leq\alpha. \end{aligned}$$

Thus, ZIP LRT method controls the type-I error when ω and p_0 are known.

The false discovery rate (FDR) is defined as the expected value of the ratio (V/R), namely, E$(\frac{\mathrm{V}}{\mathrm{R}})$, where V is the number of signals detected incorrectly, and R is the total number of signals detected. When R=0, we let $\frac{\mathrm{V}}{\mathrm{R}}$=0. Under H$_0$, $\frac{\mathrm{V}}{\mathrm{R}}$=1, for any V> 0, and

$$\mathrm{E}(\frac{\mathrm{V}}{\mathrm{R}}|\mathrm{H}_0)=1\times\mathrm{P}(\mathrm{reject\ H}_0|\mathrm{H}_0)=\alpha$$

Also, under H$_a$, $\frac{\mathrm{V}}{\mathrm{R}}\leq 1$, and

$$\begin{aligned} & \mathrm{E}(\frac{\mathrm{V}}{\mathrm{R}}|\mathrm{H}_a) \\ & =\omega\ \mathrm{E}(\frac{\mathrm{V}}{\mathrm{R}}|\mathrm{H}_a,n_{ij}\text{ is true zero})+(1-\omega)\ \mathrm{E}(\frac{\mathrm{V}}{\mathrm{R}}|\mathrm{H}_a,n_{ij}\text{ is from Poisson Model}) \\ & =0+(1-\omega)\ \mathrm{E}(\frac{\mathrm{V}}{\mathrm{R}}|\mathrm{H}_a,n_{ij}\text{ is from Poisson Model}) \\ & \leq(1-\omega)\ \mathrm{E}(\frac{\mathrm{V}}{\mathrm{R}}|\mathrm{H}_0)=(1-\omega)\alpha \end{aligned}$$

where the last inequality follows from Ref. [45]. Therefore, FDR is less than or equal to the type-I error with the adjustment of the presence of possible true zeros.

When p_0 and ω are unknown, let $\widehat{\widetilde{LR}}_{ij}$ and $\widehat{\widetilde{T}}$ be the estimates of $\widetilde{LR}_{ij}$ and $\widetilde{T}$ obtained by replacing p_0 and ω by $\hat{p}_0$ and $\hat{\omega}$. Then, we have

$$\begin{aligned} & P(|(\max_i(\widehat{\widetilde{LR}}_{ij}) - \widehat{\widetilde{T}}) - (\max_i(\widetilde{LR}_{ij}) - \widetilde{T})| > 0|H_0) \\ = \; & P(|\max_i(\widehat{\widetilde{LR}}_{ij}) - \max_i(\widetilde{LR}_{ij}) + (\widetilde{T} - \widehat{\widetilde{T}})| > 0|H_0) \\ \leq \; & P(|\max_i(\widehat{\widetilde{LR}}_{ij}) - \max_i(\widetilde{LR}_{ij})| > 0|H_0) + P(|\widehat{\widetilde{T}} - \widetilde{T}| > 0|H_0) \to 0 \end{aligned}$$

in probability since both $\widehat{\widetilde{T}}$ and $max_i \widehat{\widetilde{LR}}_{ij}$ are consistent estimators of $\widetilde{T}$ and $max_i \widetilde{LR}_{ij}$, respectively. Thus, the type-I error of $max_i \widehat{\widetilde{LR}}_{ij}$ converges in probability to that of $max_i \widetilde{LR}_{ij}$, and in the limit it is less than or equal to α. Similarly, when p_0 and ω are unknown, the false discovery rate can also be shown to be asymptotically controlled.

5.10 Tables and Figures

FIGURE 5.1
Histogram of the percentage of observed zeros for each drug (either suspect or concomitant) in the 2006–2011 data (left panel), and histogram of the estimated percentage of true zeros using EM algorithm (right panel).

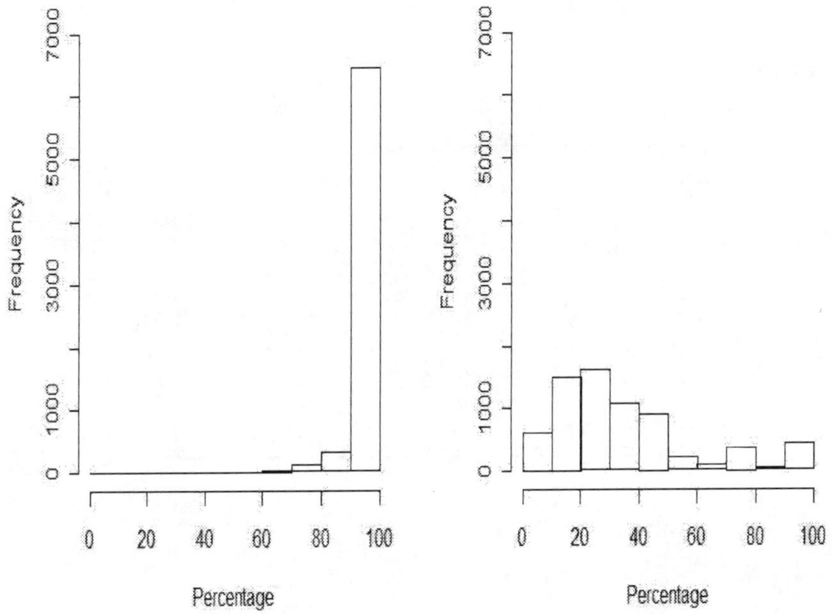

TABLE 5.1
Performance characteristics of ZIP LRT and LRT methods under $\omega = 0\%$.

Methods	$n_{.j}$	signals	η	Power(%)	ST	FDR
ZIP	12,000	0	1	3.6	-	0.0360
LRT	12,000	0	1	3.8	-	0.0380
ZIP	12,000	5	4	100	1.00	0.0089
LRT	12,000	5	4	100	1.00	0.0091

TABLE 5.2
Performance characteristics of ZIP LRT method when ω varies.

Methods	ω	$n_{.j}$	signal	η	Power(%)	ST	FDR
ZIP	0%	6,000	5	4	100	1.00	0.0082
ZIP	30%	6,000	5	4	100	0.85	0.0000
ZIP	50%	6,000	5	4	100	0.79	0.0000
ZIP	70%	6,000	5	4	100	0.79	0.0000
ZIP	90%	6,000	5	4	100	0.76	0.0000
ZIP	0%	12,000	5	4	100	1.00	0.0089
ZIP	30%	12,000	5	4	100	0.92	0.0000
ZIP	50%	12,000	5	4	100	0.90	0.0000
ZIP	70%	12,000	5	4	100	0.90	0.0000
ZIP	90%	12,000	5	4	100	0.89	0.0000

TABLE 5.3
Performance characteristic of ZIP LRT when η or $n_{.j}$ varies and $\omega = 50\%$.

$n_{.j}$	signals	η	Power(%)	ST	FDR
6,000	5	1	5	-	0.0450
6,000	5	3	75	0.17	0.0000
6,000	5	3.5	100	0.47	0.0000
6,000	5	4	100	0.79	0.0000
6,000	5	5	100	1.00	0.0000
6,000	5	6	100	1.00	0.0000
600	5	4	90	0.34	0.0037
1,000	5	3	29	0.06	0.0030
1,000	5	4	97	0.43	0.0012
3,000	5	3	45	0.10	0.0000
3,000	5	4	100	0.67	0.0003
6,000	5	4	100	0.79	0.0000
12,000	5	4	100	0.90	0.0000

TABLE 5.4
Signals (AE) detected for 6 drugs from the FAERS database for 2006–2011 data.

Drug name	$n_{.j}$	Observed zeros (%)	$\hat{\omega}$ in %	LRT	ZIP LRT
Prednisone	225,043	54.97	6.31	361	361
Aspirin	478,523	53.55	15.70	262	260
Heparin	85,797	75.94	30.84	197	165
Gadopentetic acid	17,045	93.40	64.06	113	67
Gadobenate	6,925	97.16	76.47	70	27
Docosanol	4,758	98.77	87.79	50	8

TABLE 5.5
AE signals detected for Gadobenate from the FAERS database for 2006–2011 data.

	LRT		ZIP LRT	
AE	$\log LR_{ij}$	P-value	$\log LR_{ij}$	P-value
Nephrogenic systemic fibrosis	1569.63	< .0001	1571.07	< .0001
Fibrosis	656.62	< .0001	658.06	< .0001
Hypersensitivity	494.39	< .0001	495.83	< .0001
Skin hypertrophy	443.79	< .0001	445.23	< .0001
Skin fibrosis	421.11	< .0001	422.56	< .0001
Scar	407.22	< .0001	408.67	< .0001
Skin induration	405.73	< .0001	407.18	< .0001
Mobility decreased	374.31	< .0001	375.76	< .0001
Skin tightness	355.05	< .0001	356.49	< .0001
Emotional distress	354.91	< .0001	356.36	< .0001
Pain	282.32	< .0001	283.77	< .0001
Joint contracture	280.76	< .0001	282.21	< .0001
Anaphylactoid reaction	272.28	< .0001	273.72	< .0001
Joint range of motion decreased	256.25	< .0001	257.70	< .0001
General physical health deterioration	253.23	< .0001	254.68	< .0001
Injury	198.07	< .0001	199.51	< .0001
Vomiting	177.72	< .0001	179.16	< .0001
Anxiety	171.69	< .0001	173.14	< .0001
Urticaria	168.28	< .0001	169.73	< .0001
Deformity	162.79	< .0001	164.24	< .0001
Anhedonia	150.83	< .0001	152.28	< .0001
Joint stiffness	146.06	< .0001	147.51	< .0001
Extremity contracture	138.40	< .0001	139.84	< .0001
Skin hyperpigmentation	123.87	< .0001	125.32	0.0003
Nausea	108.99	< .0001	110.44	0.0037
Skin discoloration	103.09	< .0001	104.54	0.0096
Peau d'orange	99.49	< .0001	100.93	0.0210

TABLE 5.6
Signals using gender as a covariate for two drugs from 2006–2011 FAERS data (by ZIP LRT).

	without stratification	with stratification			
Drug	Total	Total	(F)	(M)	(UN)
Gadobenate	27	29	28	26	2
Docosanol	8	15	20	5	0

Part II

Extensions

6

LRT Method for Active Safety Surveillance with Exposure Information

The earlier chapters primarily address large post-market safety data such as FAERS data with reports from insurance companies, health care professionals, patients, consumers, and other reporting resources. The exposure information in those types of data is not available or not accurate. In this chapter, we discuss a longitudinal LRT method, referred to as LongLRT [81], for the exposure-based data for active surveillance in observational or clinical trial databases for one or more drugs (such as a drug class) and/or one or more adverse events (AEs) or safety health outcomes (safety endpoints or events) of interest. This method covers the special case of Sequential LRT (SeqLRT) where the process stops at a look when a success (i.e., a signal) is found for a drug of interest vs. placebo or a comparator with a single AE of interest such as acute myocardial infarction (AMI).

6.1 Medical Background Based on the Example Data

Proton Pump Inhibitors (PPIs) are a class of drugs that decrease gastric acid secretion through inhibition of the proton pump which helps in the secretion of acid from the stomach glands. PPIs are associated with increased risk of hip fractures (side effect) [88, 145]. It is important to study the safety issues of PPIs using clinical trial datasets for regulatory labeling. Six drugs have been used as the test drugs for treating patients with osteoporosis in the clinical trials with data available from FDA/OTS/CSC legacy database.

The intention of these trials was to evaluate whether the concomitant use of PPIs reduces the efficacy of the six test drugs treating osteoporosis among targeted patients. The minimum and maximum exposure (EX) times, shown in Table 6.3, are obtained using the start date and the end date of the test drugs and placebo for individuals. The exposure information for the test drugs, including their start and end dates, is complete in the database. However, the exposure information for the concomitant use of PPIs is not complete. Additionally, a patient may have taken one or more PPI drugs with varying durations within the overall exposure period of the test drug. Therefore, we simply code the patients with concomitant PPIs having test drug as "test drug+PPIs", and the exposure time of test drug+PPIs as the exposure time of the test drug. It is expected that more AE cases associated with osteoporosis are to be observed in the subjects with concomitant PPIs. The minimum and maximum AE times (shown in Table 6.3) are, respectively, the minimum and maximum of the occurrence dates of AEs from all AEs reported in the trials.

6.1.1 Data structure

Aggregated clinical trial data with exposure information are generated from the individual-level clinical trial data. As shown in Table 6.3, ten trials from the legacy database are included in this study. Among the subjects taking a test drug for treating osteoporosis, there is a small percent of subjects concomitantly taking PPIs. Six test drugs plus placebo were used for treating female participants with postmenopausal osteoporosis and/or severe osteoporosis. The sample sizes (number of subjects) in the studies ranged from hundreds to thousands in each arm. Some patients were treated with concomitant PPIs (a single PPI or mixed use of several PPIs) during the exposure period of the test drugs. There are a total of five PPIs. The sample size of patients with concomitant PPIs in each arm is usually less than 10% of the total sample size. It is difficult to evaluate the safety issues of the concomitant use of PPIs in a single trial, as generally the study is powered for efficacy. Thus, the pooled data consisting of multiple clinical trial datasets, resulting in a large sample size, are needed for evaluating the safety issues of the concomitant use of multiple PPI drugs. The common data models, under the FDA Sentinel Initiative, have similar data structure, and hence the methodology developed can be applied to the common data models.

6.1.2 Definitions of drug exposure

We present different definitions of the drug exposure (e.g., event-time, person-time, exposure time) that can be used as a denominator for evaluating safety issues, along with different statistical models. We define all AE cases that occur during the exposure period between the start and end dates of a test drug with or without PPIs as *countable cases*. The event-time is defined as the duration from the start date of the test drug exposure to the AE (event) start date if the AE case is a *countable case*. Note that this definition of a countable case implicitly implies that all countable AE cases occur between the start and end dates of a test drug. However, there are situations, for example, in vaccine safety studies, in which the AE cases that occur 7-days after the drug exposure evaluation are defined as *countable cases*.

Each countable AE case has one event-time, and each subject can have many countable AE cases and hence many event-time records. As shown in Figure 6.1, define event-time $P_{ijs}^{l(i,s)}$ as the event-time for subject s, taking j^{th}

Drug, and having l^{th} occurrence of ith AE. Note that $P_{ijs}^{l(i,s)}$ allows for unequal event-times for different subjects. The event-time for j^{th} Drug and i^{th} AE is then the sum of the event-times of the countable cases over all subjects and occurrences, $P_{ij} = \sum_s \sum_{l(i,s)} P_{ijs}^{l(i,s)}$, where summations are over $s = 1, \cdots, S$ and $l(i,s) = 1, \cdots, L(i,s)$, respectively. S is the total number of subjects, and $L(i,s)$ is the total number of occurrences of ith AE for sth subject. The marginal row and column totals of P_{ij} are $P_{i.} = \sum_j P_{ij}$ and $P_{.j} = \sum_i P_{ij}$, and the grand total is $P_{..}$.

When each subject takes only one drug, and has a single AE reported, $L(i,s) = 1$ and $i = 1$, the event-time is exactly the person-time (shown in Figure 6.2). This is the definition used by Brown et al. [27], Li [102], and Cook et al. [32] (in active surveillance for dealing with one AE of interest and to compare a single drug vs. a comparator). If a subject does not have any AE, the person-time is simply the duration of drug exposure. The person-times for i^{th} AE and j^{th} Drug is the sum of person-times for i^{th} AE and j^{th} Drug over subjects, $P_{ij} = \sum_s P_{ijs}$.

Another way of incorporating the exposure information is to define the "exposure time", P_{ds}, for subject s taking drug d (from start date to the end date of the drug use) as the overall drug exposure duration (assuming that each subject only takes one of the 14 drugs (6 test drugs, placebo, 6 test drug+PPIs, and placebo+PPIs)). As shown in Figure 6.3, the total exposure duration for the drug d is, $P_d = \sum_s P_{ds}$, and the grand total of the exposure is $P_. = \sum_d P_d = \sum_d \sum_s P_{ds}$. Note that all AEs for subject s that occurred during P_{ds} share the same exposure duration, P_{ds}. The *countable cases* are the AE cases that occur during the "exposure time".

For subjects without any event during the drug exposure, the person-time and the exposure time are defined as the duration from the start date to the end date of the drug exposure.

6.1.3 Defining multiple looks

The analysis-period or Look k ($k = 1, \cdots, K$), includes the cumulative data from time-intervals $1, 2, \cdots$, up to kth interval, and Look K is the last look consisting of the largest analysis-period (i.e., the period containing the time-intervals $1, 2, \cdots, K$). Note that there are two ways to define the study intervals: *calendar time* and *time after treatment*. Using *calendar time* involves combining all the ten clinical studies. Unequal time-intervals 1996–97, 1998–99, 2000–01, 2002–03, and 2004–07, lead to five analysis-periods or Looks of the data defined by 1996–97, 1996–99, 1996–2001, 1996–2003, and 1996–2007. Using *time after treatment*, which is defined as the time of the first occurrence of a single AE (e.g., a composite AE consisting of all PT terms associated with osteoporosis, see details in Appendix 6.7.1) after the start of the treatment; one can evaluate the safety signal over *time after treatment* (30 days, half year, one year, etc.). However, in this chapter, only *calendar time* is considered for defining the analysis-periods.

6.2 Longitudinal LRT Method for Active Safety Surveillance

We define event rate as the ratio of the number of countable cases to the event time (as denominator). Similarly, we define risk as the ratio of the single countable case to the person-time (as denominator) or ratio of the multiple countable cases to the exposure time (as denominator).

6.2.1 LongLRT for comparing multiple events using event-time

We consider K looks ($k = 1, \cdots, K$) of the data. At Look k (i.e., kth analysis-period), let n_{ijk} be the number of countable cases for j^{th} Drug and i^{th} AE. Define, $n_{i.k} = \sum_j n_{ijk}$, $n_{.jk} = \sum_i n_{ijk}$, and $n_{..k} = \sum_i n_{i.k}$. For event-times, let P_{ijk} be the sum of event-times for j^{th} Drug and i^{th} AE, over subjects. Define, $P_{i.k} = \sum_j P_{ijk}$, $P_{.jk} = \sum_i P_{ijk}$, and $P_{..k} = \sum_i P_{i.k}$. The two $I \times J$ tables, one for the event counts and the other for event-times, with rows as AEs and columns as drugs are given in Tables 6.1 and 6.2 (shown in Appendix 6.7.2). There are I, 2×2 tables, one corresponding to each i, for event counts and event-times, respectively.

With exposure information available, assume that $n_{ijk} \sim^{ind} Poisson(p_{ijk} \times P_{i.k})$, and for other AEs combined, assume that $(n_{.jk} - n_{ijk}) \sim^{ind} Poisson(q_{ijk} \times (P_{..k} - P_{i.k}))$, where $i = 1, \cdots, I, k = 1, \cdots, K$; and where p_{ijk} and q_{ijk} are the event rates.

For fixed j and a particular look k, the test hypotheses are

$$H_0 : p_{ijk} = q_{ijk} = p_{0k}, \text{for all AE i's},$$
$$H_a : p_{ijk} > q_{ijk}, \text{for at least one AE i}.$$

Note that under H_0, the index j in p_{0k} is dropped, and $\hat{p}_{0k} = \frac{n_{.jk}}{P_{..k}}$. Under H_a, $\hat{p}_{ijk} = \frac{n_{ijk}}{P_{i.k}}$, $\hat{q}_{ijk} = \frac{n_{.jk} - n_{ijk}}{P_{..k} - P_{i.k}}$. This model evaluates relative event rate (p_{ijk}/q_{ijk}) instead of relative reporting rate by incorporating the exposure information. The relative event-rate is 1 under the null hypothesis, and > 1 under the alternative hypothesis. The signals detected are the AEs with higher relative event rate (for drug j).

The likelihood ratio (based on Poisson model) for the ith AE and fixed j^{th}

Drug is,

$$
\begin{aligned}
LR_{ijk} &= \frac{(\frac{n_{ijk}}{P_{i.k}})^{n_{ijk}}(\frac{n_{.jk}-n_{ijk}}{P_{..k}-P_{i.k}})^{n_{.jk}-n_{ijk}}}{(\frac{n_{.jk}}{P_{..k}})^{n_{.jk}}} \\
&= (\frac{n_{ijk}}{E_{ijk}})^{n_{ijk}}(\frac{n_{.jk}-n_{ijk}}{n_{.jk}-E_{ijk}})^{(n_{.jk}-n_{ijk})},
\end{aligned}
$$

where $E_{ijk} = \frac{P_{i.k} \times n_{.jk}}{P_{..k}}$. The LongLRT statistic for testing H_0 at Look k is $max_{1 \leq i \leq I} logLR_{ijk}$.

If the counts are assumed to follow independent Binomial distributions $n_{ijk} \sim^{ind} Binomial(P_{i.k}, p_{ijk})$, and $(n_{.jk} - n_{ijk}) \sim^{ind} Binomial((P_{..k} - P_{i.k}), q_{ijk})$, then the (Binomial-based) likelihood ratio for i^{th} AE and j^{th} Drug at Look k is,

$$
LR_{ijk} = \frac{(\frac{n_{ijk}}{P_{i.k}})^{n_{ijk}}(1-\frac{n_{ijk}}{P_{i.k}})^{n_{i.k}-n_{ijk}}(\frac{n_{.jk}-n_{ijk}}{P_{..k}-P_{i.k}})^{n_{.jk}-n_{ijk}}(1-\frac{n_{.jk}-n_{ijk}}{P_{..k}-P_{i.k}})^{(n_{..k}-n_{i.k})-(n_{.jk}-n_{ijk})}}{(\frac{n_{.jk}}{P_{..k}})^{n_{.jk}}(1-\frac{n_{.jk}}{P_{..k}})^{n_{..k}-n_{.jk}}}.
$$

For large $P_{i.k}(>> n_{ijk})$ and $(P_{..k} - P_{i.k})(>> (n_{.jk} - n_{ijk}))$, the Binomial-based LR_{ijk} converges to Poisson-based LR_{ijk}.

If the event-times are each one-unit time, then $P_{i.k} = n_{i.k}$ and $P_{..k} = n_{..k}$, and the LR_{ijk} becomes the likelihood ratio statistic based on spontaneous reports data discussed in Ref. [80].

LongLRT is not a regression-based approach; however, covariates can be brought in the LRT statistic through the expected counts, which are derived for the pre-specified strata as $E_{ijk} = \sum_m E_{ijk}^{(m)}$, where $E_{ijk}^{(m)} = \frac{P_{i.k}^{(m)} \times n_{.jk}^{(m)}}{P_{..k}^{(m)}}$ is the expected count for the mth stratum. The $n_{.jk}^{(m)}$, $P_{i.k}^{(m))}$, and $P_{..k}^{(m)}$ are based on the two $I \times J$ tables for $n_{ijk}^{(m)}$ and $P_{ijk}^{(m)}$ for each stratum m. Usually a limited number of factors and strata are recommended because of low sample size per stratum. In the presence of large number of covariates, propensity scores can be obtained for combining the information from the covariates if the subject-level data are available, and strata can be defined by the propensity scores.

6.2.2 SeqLRT for comparing two drugs and one AE with single occurrence using person-time

When each subject takes only one drug, either the test drug or the comparator, and has one AE event (such as death) or the first occurrence of AE such as the first occurrence of stroke or bleeding, the event-time (time from the drug exposure to the first occurrence of the AE) discussed in Section 6.2.1 is exactly the person-time (Figure 6.2).

For each k, we work with a 2×1 table, with the rows denoting the test drug and the comparator ($I = 2$), and the column as the single AE of interest ($J = 1$). Here, $P_{i.k} = P_{i1k}$, and $P_{..} = \sum_i P_{i1k} = P_{11k} + P_{21k}$. Sum of the person-times over subjects for each drug is used as the denominator, and the relative risk is evaluated.

For the AE of interest (j=1), the test hypotheses are

$$H_0 : p_{11k} = q_{21k} = p_{0k},$$
$$H_a : p_{11k} > q_{21k}.$$

Under H_0, $\hat{p}_{0k} = \frac{n_{.1k}}{P_{..k}}$ (risk of the AE of interest for the test drug and the comparator). Under H_a, $\hat{p}_{11k} = \frac{n_{11k}}{P_{1.k}} = \frac{n_{11k}}{P_{11k}}$ (risk of the AE of interest for the test drug) and $\hat{q}_{11k} = \frac{n_{.1k}-n_{11k}}{P_{..k}-P_{1.k}} = \frac{n_{21k}}{P_{21k}}$ (risk of the AE of interest for the comparator).

The likelihood ratio is

$$LR_{11k} = \frac{(\frac{n_{11k}}{P_{11k}})^{n_{11k}}(\frac{n_{21k}}{P_{21k}})^{n_{21k}}}{(\frac{n_{11k}+n_{21k}}{P_{11k}+P_{21k}})^{n_{11k}+n_{21k}}} = (\frac{n_{1k}}{E_{11k}})^{n_{11k}}(\frac{n_{21k}}{n_{.1k} - E_{11k}})^{n_{21k}},$$

where $E_{11k} = \frac{P_{11k} \times n_{.1k}}{P_{11k}+P_{21k}}$. The SeqLRT statistic for testing H_0 at Look k is $max_i logLR_{i1k}, i = 1, 2$.

This model evaluates relative risk ($RR_{11k} = p_{11k}/q_{21k}$) using person-time instead of relative event rate. The relative risk is 1, under the null hypothesis; and is greater than 1, under the alternative hypothesis. The signal detected is the drug with higher relative risk (for the AE of interest). Stratified analysis can be conducted along the same lines as discussed in Section 6.2.1.

6.2.3 LongLRT for comparing multiple drugs and one AE with recurrence using exposure-time

The methods discussed in Section 6.2.1 cannot be modified directly and applied to comparing multiple drugs using "exposure-time". In the following section, we consider a total of D drugs and J AEs (note the change in the notations), and K analysis-periods. We suppress k in the notations, and assume that each subject takes only one drug (from a total of D=14 drugs described in Section 6.1). For a fixed j (where $j*$ is a particular AE of interest or a composite AE), define P_{ds} to be the exposure time (from start date to end date) for the sth subject taking d^{th} drug ($d = 1, \cdots, D, D \geq 2$); see Figure 6.3 in which AE1, AE2, and AE3 can be treated as recurrent events for a composite AE. Let $n_{dj*s}(= \sum_l n_{dj*s}^{l(i,s)})$ be the total number of countable cases of the $j*^{th}$ AE for d^{th} drug and sth subject. In this case the $I \times J$ matrix is a $D \times 1$ matrix with rows as drugs and the single column as the AE (or the composite AE) of interest. The distribution of the events can be written as $n_{dj*s} \sim^{ind} Poisson(p_{dj*s}P_{ds})$, where p_{dj*s} is the risk of a single AE or composite AE with recurrence for sth subject.

Assuming that the risks $p_{dj*s}, s = 1, \cdots, S$ (S is the total number of subjects) are *homogeneous* over the S subjects, and denoting this common risk by p_{dj*}, we can rewrite the distribution for the events as $n_{dj*s} \sim^{ind}$

$Poisson(p_{dj*}P_{ds})$. Then, the sum of the events over all subjects, for the dth drug $n_{dj*}(=\sum_s n_{dj*s})$ follows $n_{dj*} \sim^{ind} Poisson(p_{dj*}P_d)$, where $P_d = \sum_s P_{ds}$. Note that index $j*$ is dropped from P_{ds} (and hence from P_d) because we only work with just one AE. Also, assume that the events for other drugs have the following distribution $(n_{.j*} - n_{dj*}) \sim^{ind} Poisson(q_{dj*}(P_{.} - P_d))$, where q_{dj*} is the risk (homogeneous across all subjects) for other drugs (not including d^{th} drug), $n_{.j*} = \sum_d n_{dj*}$ and $P_{.} = \sum_d P_d$ are the total number of countable cases, and the total exposure time for all drugs, respectively. The ratio $RR_{dj*} = \frac{p_{dj*}}{q_{dj*}}$ is called as the relative risk of the $j*^{th}$ AE for drug d vs. other drugs. The signals identified using this approach are the drugs with higher relative risk (for the AE of interest).

For fixed $j(j*)$, the test hypotheses are:

$$H_0 : p_{dj*} = q_{dj*} = p_0, \text{for all drug d's},$$
$$H_a : p_{dj*} > q_{dj*}, \text{for at least one drug d.}$$

Under $H_0, \hat{p}_0 = \frac{n_{.j*}}{P_{.}}$, and under $H_a, \hat{p}_{dj*} = \frac{n_{dj*}}{P_d}, \hat{q}_{dj*} = \frac{n_{.j*} - n_{d,j*}}{P_{.} - P_d}$. The likelihood ratio for d^{th} drug and fixed $j*^{th}$ AE is

$$LR_{dj*} = \frac{(\frac{n_{dj*}}{P_d})^{n_{dj*}} (\frac{n_{.j*} - n_{dj*}}{P_{.} - P_d})^{n_{.j*} - n_{dj*}}}{(\frac{n_{.j*}}{P_{.}})^{n_{.j*}}} = (\frac{n_{dj*}}{E_{dj*}})^{n_{dj*}} (\frac{n_{.j*} - n_{dj*}}{n_{.j*} - E_{dj*}})^{(n_{.j*} - n_{dj*})},$$

where $E_{dj*} = \frac{P_d \times n_{.j*}}{P_{.}}$. The maximum log likelihood ratio test statistic (LongLRT statistic) is $max_d logLR_{dj*}$.

Here, for stratified analysis, the expected counts for the pre-specified strata are given by $E_{dj*k} = \sum_m E^{(m)}_{dj*k}$, where $E^{(m)}_{dj*k} = \frac{P^{(m)}_{dk} \times n^{(m)}_{.jk}}{P^{(m)}_{.k}}$.

6.2.4 Assumption of independence

For the model described in Section 6.2.1, the assumption that the countable cases for i^{th} AE and j^{th} Drug are independent may not hold because the countable cases within one cell (i,j) and across cells could come from the same subject several times. Therefore, we relax the independence assumption for n_{ijk} and $(n_{.jk} - n_{ijk})$, $i = 1, \cdots, I$; at each fixed Look k, in the derivation of LR_{ijk} as follows:

Let $n_{ijk}|\theta \sim^{ind} Poisson(\theta p_{ijk} P_{i.k}), i = 1, \cdots, I$, and $(n_{.jk} - n_{ijk})|\theta \sim^{ind} Poisson(\theta q_{ij}(P_{..k} - P_{i.k})), i = 1, \cdots, I$, where $\theta \sim Gamma(1, 1)$, with both the scale and shape parameters equal to 1, and with pdf $g(\theta|1, 1)$. Then, it can be shown that (dropping indexes k):

$$E(n_{ij}) = P_{i.} p_{ij}, Var(n_{ij}) = P_{i.} p_{ij}(1 + P_{i.} p_{ij})$$

and

$$Cov(n_{ij}, n_{i'j}) = (P_{i.} p_{ij}) \times (P_{i'.} p_{i'j}),$$

so that

$$0 < Corr(n_{ij}, n_{i'j}) = \sqrt{\frac{(P_{i.}p_{ij}) \times (P_{i'.}p_{i'j})}{(1 + P_{i.}p_{ij}) \times (1 + P_{i'.}p_{i'j})}} < 1.$$

As shown in the Appendix 6.7.3, the expression for the likelihood ratio LR_{ij} is unaffected at any look k, and the conditional distribution of $(n_{1jk}, \cdots, n_{Ijk})$, given $n_{.jk}$ under H_0, is still $Multinomial(n_{.jk}, (\frac{P_{1.k}}{P_{..k}}, \cdots, \frac{P_{I.k}}{P_{..k}}))$, independent of θ. This shows the robustness of LRT performance for data with or without correlation. However, the serial dependence of n_{ijk} through an autocorrelation between n_{ijk} and $n_{ijk'}(k < k')$ needs to be investigated.

6.3 Statistical Inference with Multiple Looks

Since the asymptotic distribution of the LongLRT statistic is analytically not tractable, the Monte Carlo approach is used to obtain the empirical distribution. For the test statistics discussed in Sections 6.2.1 and 6.2.2, the joint distribution of the cell counts is given by

$$(n_{1jk}, \cdots, n_{Ijk})|n_{.jk} \sim Multinomial(n_{.jk}, (\frac{P_{1.k}}{P_{..k}}, \cdots, \frac{P_{I.k}}{P_{..k}})),$$

where I is the total number of rows. For the test statistic discussed in Section 6.2.3, the joint distribution of the cell counts is given by

$$(n_{1j*k}, \cdots, n_{Dj*k})|n_{.j*k} \sim Multinomial(n_{.j*k}, (\frac{P_{1k}}{P_{.k}}, \cdots, \frac{P_{Dk}}{P_{.k}})),$$

where D is the total number of drugs under comparison. The totals $n_{.jk}$, $P_{i.k}$, $P_{..k}$, n_{dj*k}, P_{dk} and $P_{.k}$ are from the observed data and are fixed in the simulation for p-value calculation.

The values of the test statistic $max_{1 \leq i \leq I} logLR_{ijk}$ are calculated for the observed dataset and 9,999 simulated null datasets, and are used to derive the empirical distribution. At each Look k, we test the hypothesis H_0 vs. H_a, with level of significance $\alpha(k)$ specified.

We can use an increasing α-spending function [84, 102], given by $\alpha(k) = \frac{1}{K}\alpha, k = 1, \cdots, K$ with $\alpha(0) = 0$, so that cumulative error $\alpha^*(k) = \frac{k}{K}\alpha \leq \alpha$, or a decreasing α-spending function (proposed by Goodman et al. [57]), given by $\alpha(k) = \frac{\alpha}{2^k}$ so that cumulative error $\alpha^*(k) = \alpha \sum_{r=1}^{k} \frac{1}{2^r} \leq \alpha$. If α is specified as 0.05, the cumulative error at kth look is always less than 0.05 for both functions. The advantage of the decreasing spending function is that one does not need to specify K, the maximum number of looks. Other α-spending functions, incorporating the fraction of information used, can also be considered [101, 117].

A signal is found if the observed $max_i logLR_{ijk}$ from the real data is greater than the $100(1-\alpha(k))\%$ cut-off point of the empirical distribution of the $max_i logLR_{ijk}$ under H_0. We use step-down procedure to identify the secondary, tertiary, and other lower order signals.

The proposed LongLRT method controls (family-wise) type-I error, α, in two ways: first, it controls alpha across the pre-specified number of looks of the data using a monotone alpha-spending function; and then, at each look, it controls the fraction of alpha assigned at that look for multiplicity by using the step-down procedure for testing multiple hypotheses for potential signals. The LongLRT method also controls the false discovery rate (FDR) with FDR $\leq \alpha$ (for details, see Ref. [80]).

6.4 Applications

In the following section, we present the results from the applications of LongLRT and SeqLRT discussed in Sections 6.2 and 6.3 to the pooled clinical trial data with exposure information for detecting AE signals for a drug, or for detecting drug signals for the composite AE associated with osteoporosis (AEOST). The SeqLRT and LongLRT with Poisson and Binomial models provide similar results in applications. Therefore, only results for Poisson model are presented here.

We use $\alpha = 0.05$ and decreasing alpha-spending function, as it helps to detect more signals early on, in a short duration, and subsequently get the confirmation of the detected signals with more data (with smaller α).

At Look k, if the p-value for an AE from the LongLRT method is less than $\alpha(k) = \frac{\alpha}{2^k}$ (with $\alpha(1) = 0.025, \alpha(2) = 0.0125, \alpha(3) = 0.00625, \alpha(4) = 0.003125, \alpha(5) = 0.001563$), then that the ith AE is a signal. Once a signal is identified, the search process can be stopped. However, it is continued for signal confirmation or refinement. For example, a signal detected at Look $k = 2$ may not more be a signal at Look k=3. In that case, the signal detected at Look $k = 2$ is not confirmed.

Note that there are approximately 10% patients with concomitant use of PPIs in this clinical trial database. The prevalence of PPI use likely has an effect on the number of the observed AEs, which in turn may affect the power of the test.

6.4.1 Safety signals (among multiple AEs) by drug

The AE signals are explored by comparing all AEs by drug in the pooled clinical trial database (1996–2007) including 14 drugs (6 test drugs, placebo, 6 test drugs+PPIs, placebo+PPIs), over 5 cumulative analysis-periods (1996–97, –99, –2001, –03, and –07). The LongLRT model discussed in Section 6.2.1

is applied here. Event-time defined as duration from the start of the drug exposure to any of the AE events is evaluated. The AEs with higher relative event rates are reported as signals.

Because of the space limitation, results for only 6 drugs (not for all 14 drugs) are presented in Table 6.4. The table gives "ndotj" as the total number of countable cases for a particular drug j; number of AE signals; selected AE signals (with relative event rate, RR) related to osteoporosis. As some drugs are used only in some trials conducted in later periods (k=3, 4, and 5), AE data for those drugs in the two earlier periods does not exist. Placebo (PL) AE data for all the five periods (k=1 to 5) is available. Some AE signals associated with osteoporosis are detected for all 14 drugs. The relative event rates for these AE signals are usually high for the drug+PPIs groups.

In the following sub-sections, we illustrate exploring the composite AE, AEOST, which is further defined in Appendix 6.7.1.

6.4.2 Safety signals for the first occurrence of a composite AE and two drugs using SeqLRT

The SeqLRT (discussed in Section 6.2.2) is applied to the pooled clinical trial data at the first occurrence of the single composite AE, AEOST, and for comparing Placebo vs. Placebo+PPIs. Once the 1st occurrence of AEOST is detected as a signal in the kth analysis-period, we stop the process of searching for safety signals in the (k+1)th analysis-periods. Each subject has only one event, if any. The event-time defined as the duration from the start of the drug exposure to the 1st occurrence of the event (or to the end of drug exposure if there is no countable event) is the person-time for each subject. The relative risk of the 1st occurrence of AEOST is evaluated in this application.

The sample sizes ($n_{.j}$), for AEOST, are 57, 163, 232, 439, and 500 for analysis-periods 1, 2, 3, 4, and 5, respectively. The relative risks of Placebo+PPIs vs. Placebo are 4.7, 2.4, 2.5, 1.9, and 1.7, for analysis-periods 1, 2, 3, 4, and 5, respectively. When $k = 1$, the p-value is 0.001 ($< \alpha(1) = 0.025$). The relative risk of AEOST for Placebo+PPIs vs. Placebo is significant at the 1st analysis-period. Therefore, we chose to stop the search for detecting further signals by the sequential method.

6.4.3 Safety signals for multiple occurrences of a composite AE and two drugs using LongLRT

The LongLRT (discussed in Section 6.2.3) is applied to the data for the single composite AE, AEOST, with recurrence, and for comparing pair of drugs (test drug+PPIs vs. test drug, or placebo+PPIs vs. placebo). In order to evaluate the relative risk of any occurrence of AEOST, the exposure time instead of event-time is used. The exposure time is defined as the duration from the start of a drug d exposure to the end of the drug d exposure for a subject s, P_{ds}.

In Table 6.5, "ndotj" is the total number of countable cases of the composite AE for the two drugs for comparison (drug and drug+PPIs), RR is the relative risk of a drug+PPIs vs. the drug. As shown in Table 6.5, the placebo+PPIs group has a higher relative risk of AEOST (with RR 2 to 6) than the placebo group over the five analysis-periods.

After the first analysis period, the relative risk (RR 1.2 to 6) is higher for all drug+PPIs than the drug only groups. In addition to the placebo+PPIs, Bazedoxifene+PPIs and LASO+PPIs also have significant AEOST signals detected at k=4 and 5 (RR 1.2 to 3).

Note that the sample sizes for AEOST for placebo+PPIs vs. placebo in Table 6.5 are larger than the corresponding sample sizes given in Section 6.4.2 because the reoccurrences of AEOST are counted and added for the analyses.

6.4.4 Safety signals for a composite AE with recurrence from multiple drugs using LongLRT

Here, we apply the LongLRT to the 14 drugs in the clinical trial database with the composite AE, AEOST. In Table 6.6, AEOST is a signal when the p-values are in "bold" (i.e., p-values $< \alpha(k)$), and RR is the relative risk of one drug vs. the other 13 drugs.

AEOST appears to be a signal for Lasoxifene, Lasoxifene+PPIs, PTH, PTH+PPIs, and Bazedoxifene+PPIs for some periods in addition to being a signal with high risk for placebo+PPIs for all the five analysis-periods. The patients in the placebo+PPIs group are not treated with drugs for osteoporosis, but with some PPIs. The high risks with significant p-values across all the analysis-periods for placebo+PPIs indicate a possible relationship between PPIs and the composite AE, AEOST.

6.5 Simulation Study for Longitudinal LRT Methods

A simulation study for evaluating the performance characteristics of proposed methods may offer a better understanding of correctly identifying the signals.

The simulation study focuses on (i) the SeqLRT using person-time for the 1st occurrence of AEOST, and (ii) the LongLRT using exposure-time for the recurrence of AEOST for the two drugs Placebo(PL)+PPIs vs. Placebo (PL). The power and type-I error are obtained.

6.5.1 Data simulation

Consider the simple case of comparing PL (i=1) and PL+PPIs (i=2). The AE of interest is the 1st occurrence of AEOST (j=1). We use the person-time (P_{i1k}) and cell counts (n_{i1k}) from the real data, and obtain $P_{i.k} = P_{i1k}, n_{.1k} = \sum_i n_{i1k}, P_{..k} = \sum_i P_{i1k}$ over the cumulative analysis-periods

($k = 1, \cdots, 5$). The cases n_{i1k} are simulated from the Binomial distribution, $n_{i1k}|n_{.1k} \sim Binomial(n_{.1k}, \frac{\eta_{i1k}P_{i.k}}{\eta_{i1k}P_{i.k}+(P_{..k}-P_{i.k})})$, where $i = 1, I(=2)$. Note that the Binomial probability of an AE depends on η (unknown) and the event-times $P_{i.k}$ and $P_{..k}$ (obtained from the real data). The SeqLRT method is applied to this simulated data.

Similarly, using the exposure-time (P_d) and cell counts (n_{ij}) from the real data, we simulate

$$(n_{1jk}, \cdots, n_{Djk})|n_{.jk} \sim Multinomial(n_{.jk}, (\eta_{1j}r_0\frac{P_{1k}}{P_{.k}}, \cdots, \eta_{Dj}r_0\frac{P_{Dk}}{P_{.k}})), \tag{6.1}$$

where r_0 is the baseline risk, which may vary in different datasets; $P_{.k} = \sum_d P_{dk}$, $\eta_{dj} \geq 1$, and $\sum_{d=1}^{D} \eta_{dj}rr_0\frac{P_{dk}}{P_{.k}} = 1; andj = 1$. This simulation process is similar to the process used in the basic LRT method simulation study (Equation 3.4). The relative risk of PL+PPIs vs. PL is η_{21}/η_{11} when $I = 2$ or $D = 2$.

For generating the data under the null hypothesis, we set $\eta_{i1} = 1$ for $i = 1, 2$, and under the alternative hypothesis, we set $\eta_{11} = 1$ (PL) and $\eta_{21} = c > 1$ (PL+PPIs) for all five analysis-periods (c values could be constant, decreasing, or increasing, over looks) assuming that the signal exists in some periods. M(=1000) datasets are simulated with different c values (1.2, 1.5, 2, 4). To evaluate the effect of sample size, we define the sample size as $z \times n_{.1k}$, where $z = 0.5, 1, 2, 4$, and z is 1 for all cases with varying c values over time.

6.5.2 Performance characteristics

Define the probability of rejecting H_0 at analysis-period k as

$$pr(k) = \frac{\#\text{rejecting } H_0 \text{ at kth period}}{1000}, k = 1, \cdots, 5.$$

This is the conditional power of the LongLRT at analysis-period k.

For the SeqLRT method with person-time generated under H_a, the probability of rejecting H_0 at analysis-period k is the sum of the probabilities of rejecting H_0 from analysis-periods 1 through k:

$$power(k) = pr(1) + \cdots + (1 - pr(1)) \times \cdots \times (1 - pr(k-1)) \times pr(k).$$

This is the unconditional power of the SeqLRT at analysis-period k.

In case of data generated under H_0, $pr(k)$ is the conditional type-I error rate for the kth analysis-period, and the values of $power(k)$ become type-I error for the SeqLRT. Without stopping the procedure, the cumulative error rate (cumer(k)) for the LongLRT is the sum of probabilities of rejecting H_0 when H_0 is true.

6.5.3 Simulation results

In this section, we present the conditional power, conditional type-I error rate, and the cumulative error rate for the LongLRT; power, type-I error, and the unconditional error rate for the SeqLRT are presented in Tables 6.7 and 6.8.

As shown in Table 6.7 with constant η values for the five periods, the power for the SeqLRT is large for the later analysis-periods, for large sample sizes, and for higher relative risk (RR) values. The simulation study shows that at the analysis period 1, the power is 0.75 for z=1 (i.e., sample size of the simulated data is equal to the sample size of the real data) and $RR = 4$ (Placebo+PPIs vs. Placebo). This result supports the finding from the real data analysis.

Additionally, the cumulative error rate of the LongLRT (shown in Table 6.7) is close to $\alpha \sum_{r=1}^{k} \frac{1}{2^r}$ level for each analysis-period. Similar patterns on the error rates are observed when the increasing α-spending function ($\alpha(k) = \frac{k}{K}\alpha$ with $K = 5$) is used (results not shown).

Table 6.8 provides the simulation results with varying RR values over time. The results show that the conditional power of both, the SeqLRT and LongLRT, have increasing (decreasing) patterns with increasing (decreasing) RR values. The unconditional power of SeqLRT increases over all five looks and approaches 1 at Look 5.

6.6 Discussion

The longitudinal LRT methodology presented here covers handling of data from a clinical trial or from administrative/claims databases with different types of exposure information. The proposed methods can be used in active surveillance for signal detection or signal generation, signal refinement, and signal validation. One of the advantages of the LongLRT methods presented here is that the methods can be used to find signals of multiple AEs (or drugs) in real-time, while controlling the FDR and the type-I error assigned at each look or across the looks. Another advantage of these methods is that one does not have to stop the analysis after a signal is detected at a look. Therefore, the number of looks for the LongLRT methods is usually not pre-specified thus providing the user more flexibility

In the special case with two drugs (e.g., Placebo and Placebo+PPIs) and a single AE, the SeqLRT evaluates the same relative risk that is evaluated by the conditional sequential sampling plan (CSSP) method proposed by Li [102]. There is a difference in the two test statistics: the SeqLRT statistic is the likelihood ratio test statistic defined as maxLR=max(LR_{11k}, LR_{21k}), see Section 6.2.2, whereas the CSSP statistic [102] is the number of AEs from the drug conditional on the total number of events from the drug and comparator;

that is, $T_{11k} = n_{11k}|n_{.1k}(= n_{11k} + n_{21k})$. However, the null data simulation process for the CSSP is the same as that proposed for the SeqLRT method with exposure data: Under H_0, $n_{11k}|n_{.1k} \sim Binomial(n_{.1k}, \frac{P_{11k}}{P_{11k}+P_{21k}})$. For a given AE of interest, if a signal is detected at a look k using the SeqLRT method, then that signal is either the drug signal or the placebo/comparator signal. However, for a given AE, if a signal is detected at look k using the CSSP method, then that signal is the drug signal only. We applied the CSSP method to the example in Section 6.4.2 (for a single AE event) and noticed that the results were the same as that from the SeqLRT (PLandPPI detected as drug signal) at the same significance level. In addition, by a simulation exploration using the set-up described in Section 6.4, we observed that both the SeqLRT and CSSP methods control the type-I error, and both have comparable power (results not shown).

The Binomial maxSPRT method, developed by Lieu et al. [104] for vaccine safety data surveillance, is a special case of the SeqLRT as shown below. It considers the exposure matching ($P_{1.k} : P_{..k}$) in a fixed matching ratio form (1:M+1). Let $n_{.k} = n_{.1k}$ be the total number of cases exposed up to time-interval k, and let $n_k^{drug} = n_{11k}$ be the number of cases exposed to the drug. Then, $E_{11k} = \frac{n_{.k}\times P_{1.k}}{P_{..k}} = \frac{n_{.k}\times 1}{M+1} = \frac{n_{.k}}{M+1}$, and the LRT_{11k}, based on Poisson model discussed in Section 6.2, can be re-written as

$$LRT_k = [(\frac{n_k^{drug}}{n_{.k}})^{n_k^{drug}}(\frac{n_{.k} - n_k^{drug}}{n_{.k}})^{n_{.k}-n_k^{drug}}]/[(\frac{1}{M+1})^{n_k^{drug}}(\frac{M}{M+1})^{n_{.k}-n_k^{drug}}],$$

which is the Binomial maxSPRT [104]).

The proposed longLRT methods with exposure unit 1 (Section 6.2) can also be used for count data collected through spontaneous systems. We explored the AE signals for the five PPIs and three test drugs, approved in US (Raloxifene, Teriparatide, and Ibandronate), in the whole FAERS database (2000–2009) over 6 analysis periods (2000–04, –05, –06, –07, –08, –09). Since the exposure information is limited in the FAERS data, only counts and relative reporting rates were evaluated. We found that very few AE signals were detected among the PPI drugs. However, many AE signals including some AEs associated with osteoporosis such as Bone density decreased, Bone pain, and Muscle spasms were detected for the three drugs for treating osteoporosis (Raloxifene, Teriparatide, and Ibandronate). It is possible that the patients with the symptoms of osteoporosis (taking the treatment drugs) reported the symptoms of osteoporosis as AEs in the FAERS data. This reveals a common problem in these types of databases that the drug products for treating a disease are reported to be associated with the symptoms of that disease.

The ZIP LRT method presented in Chapter 5 can be extended to analyze the longitudinal post-market safety data collected over time. If the database has exposure information, the ZIP model can be modified as follows. Following the notations in Section 6.2, let n_{ijk} and P_{ijk} be the number of reported cell-counts and the total exposure for the ith AE, j^{th} Drug and at kth look (i.e., at the kth analysis period). Let $n_{i.k}$ and $n_{.jk}$ be defined as the total number cell report counts for the ith AE and for the jth Drug, respectively, and let $n_{..k}$ denote the grand total of the reports at look k. Define $P_{i.k}$, $P_{.jk}$, and $P_{..k}$ similarly. Assuming that $n_{ijk} \sim Poisson(P_{i.k} \times p_{ijk})$, and $(n_{.jk} - n_{ijk}) \sim Poisson((P_{..k} - P_{i.k}) \times q_{ijk})$, the LRT test statistic at look k takes the same form as before with E_{ij} replaced by $E_{ijk} = \frac{P_{i.k} \times n_{.jk}}{P_{..k}}$. The ZIP LRT for longitudinal data with exposure information can be modeled by assuming n_{ijk} is either a true zero with probability ω_{jk}, or is a Poisson modeled count, $Poisson(P_{ijk} \times p_{ijk})$, with probability $(1 - \omega_{jk})$. The EM algorithm can be applied to the data accumulated at each look k to estimate the true zero probability ω_{jk}, p_{ijk} and the q_{ijk} under both the null and alternative hypotheses.

A monotone (increasing or decreasing) alpha spending function assigns the alpha-value to each look, so that the overall type-I error is controlled and can be used to evaluate the threshold at each look k. The ZIP LRT can also be applied to large clinical trial safety dataset, with multiple drugs and multiple AEs, where there is a possibility of high percentage of zero cells, with or without exposure information.

Because the safety data analyzed in this chapter are obtained from clinical trials, the under-reporting (or over-reporting) is not a serious concern. A stratified analysis can be used if the information on severity, disease status, and other covariates is available. In observational safety databases, the spontaneous reports can be subject to under-reporting (or over-reporting). Models can be developed along the lines of Clegg et al. [31] and Midthune et al. [108] to address this delay or error in reporting the AEs.

6.7 Appendix

6.7.1 Definition of the composite AE

The composite AE related with osteoporosis symptoms is defined as AEOST, including the following AE terms appeared in the ten clinical trial datasets: "BONE FRACTURE ACCIDENTAL", "BONE PAIN", "Bone pain", "Bone density decreased"; "MUSCLE ATROPHY", "MUSCLE CRAMP", "MUSCLE CRAMPS", "MUSCLE SPASMS", "Muscle cramp", "Muscle rupture", "Muscle spasms", "Muscle strain", "MUSCULOSKELETAL PAIN", "Musculoskeletal pain"; "JOINT SPRAIN", "JOINT STIFFNESS", "Joint contracture", "Joint crepitation", "Joint injury", "Joint sprain", "Joint stiffness"; "OSTEOPOROSIS", "OSTEOPOROSIS FRACTU", "OSTEOPOROSIS FRACTURE", "Osteoporosis"; "ANKLE FRACTURE", "Ankle fracture", "Clavicle fracture", "FOOT FRACTURE", "Facial bones fracture", "Femoral neck fracture", "Femur fracture", "Fibula fracture", "Foot fracture", "Fracture", "HUMERUS FRACTURE", "Hand fracture", "Hip fracture", "Humerus fracture", "Lower limb fracture", "Lumbar vertebral fracture", "OSTEOPOROSIS FRACTURE", "PATHOLOGICAL FRACTURE", "Patella fracture", "Pelvic fracture", "RIB FRACTURE", "Radius fracture", "Rib fracture", "SPINAL FRACTURE", "STRESS FRACTURE", "Sternal fracture", "Tibia fracture", "Ulna fracture", "Upper limb fracture", "WRIST FRACTURE" and "Wrist fracture".

6.7.2 Data structure for the $I \times J$ matrix

At look $k (k = 1, \ldots, K = 5)$, there are two $I \times J$ tables (Tables 6.1 and 6.2) constructed from the individual level data (discussed in Section 6.2.1). n_{ij} is the events for the ith AE and j^{th} Drug. P_{ij} is the event-time (with "day" as the unit) for the ith AE and j^{th} Drug. We suppress k in the notation. The row represents AE, and column represents drug.

TABLE 6.1
$I \times J$ table with event information.

AE	Drug					
	1	$\cdots$	j	$\cdots$	$J = 14$	row total
1	n_{11}	$\cdots$	n_{1j}	$\cdots$	n_{1J}	$n_{1.}$
2	n_{21}	$\cdots$	$\cdots$	$\cdots$	n_{2J}	$n_{2.}$
$\cdots$	$\cdots$	$\cdots$	$\cdots$	$\cdots$	$\cdots$	$\cdots$
i	$\cdots$	$\cdots$	n_{ij}	$\cdots$	n_{iJ}	$n_{i.}$
$\cdots$	$\cdots$	$\cdots$	$\cdots$	$\cdots$	$\cdots$	$\cdots$
I	n_{I1}	$\cdots$	n_{Ij}	$\cdots$	n_{IJ}	$n_{I.}$
column total	$n_{.1}$	$\cdots$	$n_{.j}$	$\cdots$	$n_{.J}$	$n_{..}$ as grand total

TABLE 6.2
$I \times J$ table incorporating exposure information.

AE	Drug					
	1	$\cdots$	j	$\cdots$	$J = 14$	row total
1	P_{11}	$\cdots$	P_{1j}	$\cdots$	P_{1J}	$P_{1.}$
2	P_{21}	$\cdots$	$\cdots$	$\cdots$	P_{2J}	$P_{2.}$
$\cdots$	$\cdots$	$\cdots$	$\cdots$	$\cdots$	$\cdots$	$\cdots$
i	$\cdots$	$\cdots$	P_{ij}	$\cdots$	P_{iJ}	$P_{i.}$
$\cdots$	$\cdots$	$\cdots$	$\cdots$	$\cdots$	$\cdots$	$\cdots$
I	P_{I1}	$\cdots$	P_{Ij}	$\cdots$	P_{IJ}	$P_{I.}$
column total	$P_{.1}$	$\cdots$	$P_{.j}$	$\cdots$	$P_{.J}$	$P_{..}$ as grand total

6.7.3 Independence of the parameters

Dropping the indexes j and k whenever convenient, and assuming that

$$1)\ \ n_{ij}|\theta \sim^{ind} Poisson(\theta p_i P_{i.}), i = 1, \cdots, I$$

$$2)\ \ (n_{.j} - n_{ij})|\theta \sim^{ind} (\theta q_i(P_{..} - P_{i.}), i = 1, \cdots, I$$

$$3)\ \ \theta \sim Gamma(1, 1)$$

leads to marginal (integrated) likelihood function under $H_0 : p_i = q - i = p_0, \forall i$, as

$$L_{0,ij} \propto \int_0^\infty P(n_{ij}|\theta p_i P_{i.})P(n_{.j} - n_{ij}|\theta q_i(P_{..} - Pi.))g(\theta|1, 1)d\theta,$$

where $P(x|\lambda)$ is the Poisson probability mass function, and $g(\theta|1, 1)$ is the pdf of $Gamma(.|1, 1)$.

Simplifying, we get

$$L_{0,ij}(p_0) \propto \frac{p_0^{n_{ij}}}{(1 + P_{..}p_0)^{n_{.j}+1}}$$

or

$$log[L_{ij}(p_0)] \propto n_{ij}ln(p_0) + (n_{.j} + 1)log(1 + P_{..}p_0)$$

and differentiating with reference to p_0 gives p_0 as $\hat{p}_0 = \frac{n_{.j}}{P_{..}}$.

Also, under two-sided alternative, $H_a^* : p_i \neq q_i$ for at least one i, the marginal likelihood function is

$$L_{0,ij}(p_i, q_i) \propto \frac{p_i^{n_{ij}} q_i^{n_{.j}-n_{ij}}}{(1 + P_{i.}p_i + (P_{..} - P_{i.})q_i)^{n_{.j}+1}}$$

or

$$l_{a,ij} = logL_{a,ij} \propto n_{ij}ln(p_i) + (n_{.j} - n_{ij})ln(q_i) - (n_{.j} + 1)ln(1 + p_iP_{i.} + (q_i(P_{..} - P_{i.})),$$

so that

$$\frac{\partial l_{a,ij}}{\partial p_i} = 0 \Rightarrow \frac{n_{ij}}{p_i} - \frac{(n_{.j} + 1)}{(1 + p_iP_{i.} + q_i(P_{..} - P_{i.}))} = 0$$
$$\frac{\partial l_{a,ij}}{\partial q_i} = 0 \Rightarrow \frac{n_{.j} - n_{ij}}{q_i} - \frac{(n_{.j} + 1)}{(1 + p_iP_{i.} + q_i(P_{..} - P_{i.}))} = 0.$$

Solving these equations, yield: $\hat{p}_i = \frac{n_{ij}}{P_{i.}}$, and $\hat{q}_i = \frac{n_{.j}-n_{ij}}{P_{..}-P_{i.}}$. Substituting these estimates in $L_{0,ij}$ and $L_{a,ij}$, and simplifying, we get

$$L_{ij} = \frac{L_{a,ij}(\hat{p}_i, \hat{q}_i)}{L_{0,ij}(\hat{p}_0)} = (n_{ij}/E_{ij})^{n_{ij}}((n_{.j} - n_{ij})/(n_{.j} - E_{ij}))^{n_{.j}-n_{ij}},$$

with $E_{ij} = \frac{P_{i.} \times n_{.j}}{P_{..}}$, independent of θ.

6.8 Tables and Figures

FIGURE 6.1
Definition of event-time. * is the start date of drug j and ** is the stop date of drug j. Circled dots are the occurrences of AEs (AE i, $i = 1, 2, 3, \cdots$). Only AEs between * and ** are *countable* cases and are shown in the plots over time. P^1_{ijs} is the event-time for sth subject taking j^{th} Drug with 1st occurrence of ith AE. P^2_{ijs} is the event-time for sth subject taking j^{th} Drug with 2nd occurrence of ith AE.

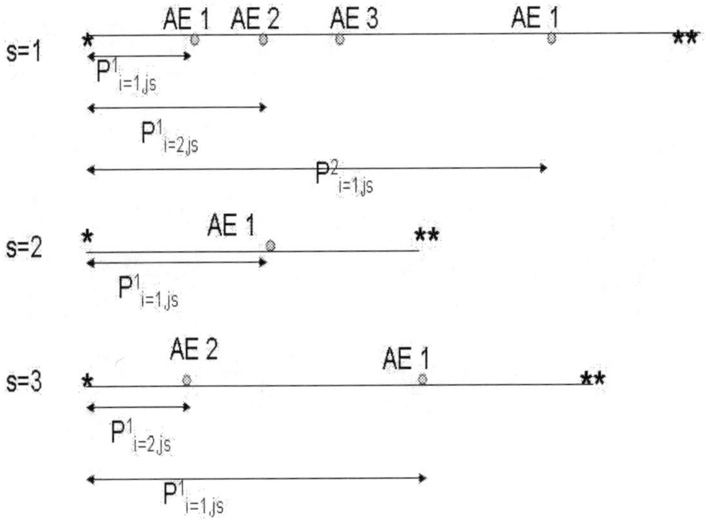

FIGURE 6.2
Definition of person-time. * is the start date of drug j and ** is the stop date of drug j. Circled dots are the occurrences of AEs (AE 1 is the AE of interest). Only AE1 between * and ** are *countable* cases and are shown in the plots over time. $P_{1js} = P^1_{1js}$ is the event-time for sth subject taking j^{th} Drug with 1st occurrence of ith AE1, which is also person-time.

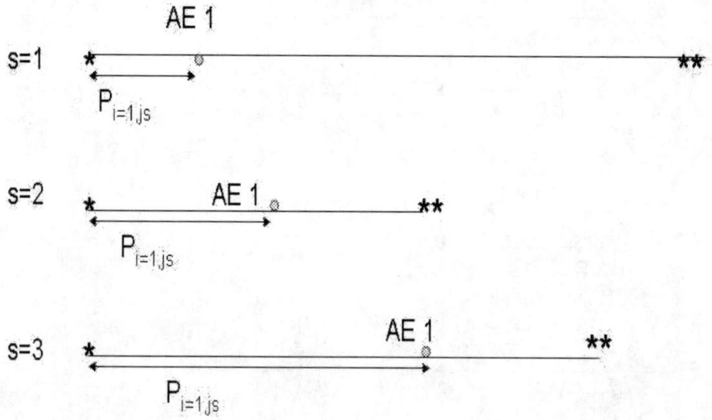

TABLE 6.3
Summary information of the clinical trials for PPIs in the legacy database.

Trials	Test drug for treating Osteoporosis		Concomitant PPIs		EX time		AE time	
	Test drug	N(subject)	# PPI drugs	N(subject)	min	max	min	max
Trial 1	Bazedoxifene	1025	5	71	2001	2004	1983	2014
	Placebo	334	5	25				
	Raloxifene	332	5	29				
Trial 2	Bazedoxifene	3778	5	477	2001	2007	1947	2006
	Placebo	1892	5	245				
	Raloxifene	1856	5	302				
Trial 3	Lasofoxifene	8556	5	965	2001	2006	2000	2006
Trial 4	Lasofoxifene	685	5	64	2000	2003	2000	2003
	Placebo	230	4	20				
Trial 5	Lasofoxifene	734	5	60	2000	2003	2000	2003
	Placebo	245	5	36				
Trial 6	PTH	1261	5	176	2000	2003	2000	2003
	Placebo	1223	5	165				
Trial 7	Teriparatide	1093	3	38	1996	1999	1920	2019
	Placebo	544	3	19				
Trial 8	Teriparatide	289	3	12	1997	1999	1920	1999
	Placebo	147	0	0				
Trial 9	Ibandronate	1964	4	82	1996	2000	1996	2000
	Placebo	982	3	32				
Trial 10	Ibandronate	489	3	21	1998	2001	1998	2001
	Placebo	159	3	9				

FIGURE 6.3
Definition of exposure-time. * is the start date of drug d and ** is the stop date of drug d. Circled dots are the occurrence of AEs (AE i, $i = 1, 2, 3, \cdots$). Only AEs between * and ** (exposure duration) are *countable* cases and are shown in the plots over time. P_{ds} is the exposure-time for sth subject taking d^{th} drug with multiple AEs during the exposure duration.

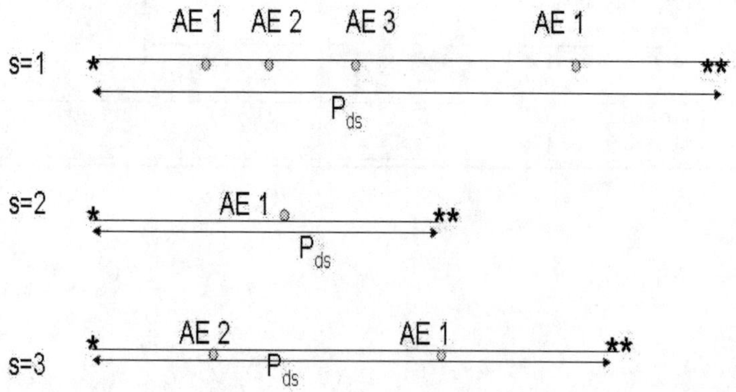

TABLE 6.4
AE signals detected by drug for the pooled clinical trial data (1996–2007) with 14 drugs.

		k=1	2	3	4	5
Placebo	ndotj	1251	4703	8282	29731	50364
	AE signals	3	6	34	43	74
	Muscle cramp (RR)			4.1	2.3	4.4
	Bone pain (RR)					2.2
Placebo+PPIs	ndotj	95	273	1094	4833	9043
	AE signals	0	0	23	26	30
	Muscle cramp (RR)					6.8
	Muscle spasms (RR)					3.9
Bazedoxifene	ndotj			516	34234	74032
	AE signals			16	115	115
	Muscle cramp (RR)				3.1	2.5
Bazedoxifene+PPIs	ndotj			846	5760	13721
	AE signals			6	53	61
	Muscle cramp (RR)				6	2.4
	Muscle spasms (RR)				6.2	4.8
PTH	ndotj			2938	9538	9538
	AE signals			89	73	114
	Joint sprain (RR)				3.1	4
	Muscle spasms (RR)			11.6		
	Muscle cramp (RR)			16.6	8.3	27.1
PTH+PPIs	ndotj			677	1724	1724
	AE signals			35	20	36
	Foot fracture (RR)					10.5
	Muscle cramp (RR)			22	9.4	30.5
	Bone pain (RR)			47.8		

Relative reporting rate (RR) values are presented when AE is detected as a signal for a particular period (p-value$< \alpha(k) = \alpha/(2^k)$).

TABLE 6.5
The composite AEOST and two drug comparison for 7 drug pairs.

		k=1	2	3	4	5
Placebo+PPIs vs. Placebo	ndotj	65	195	286	647	787
	RR	5.7	3.2	2.9	2.5	2.4
	pvalue	**0**	**0**	**0**	**0**	**0**
Ibandronate+PPIs vs. Ibandronate	ndotj	105	338	385	385	385
	RR	1.3	1.3	1.4	1.4	1.4
	pvalue	0.50	0.34	0.15	0.15	0.15
Teriparatide+PPIs vs. Teriparatide	ndotj	4	16	16	16	16
	RR		4	4	4	4
	pvalue		0.07	0.07	0.07	0.07
Raloxifene+PPIs vs. Raloxifene	ndotj			4	157	313
	RR			3.2	1.1	1.2
	pvalue			0.14	0.66	0.38
PTH+PPIs vs. PTH	ndotj			86	249	249
	RR			1.6	1.4	1.4
	pvalue			0.09	0.09	0.09
Bazedoxifene+PPIs vs. Bazedoxifene	ndotj			2	343	648
	RR				2.8	1.6
	pvalue				**0**	**0**
Lasoxifene+PPIs vs. Lasoxifene	ndotj			36	2105	3643
	RR			2.4	1.4	1.4
	pvalue			0.0385	**0**	**0**

TABLE 6.6
Single AE (the composite AEOST) and multiple drugs (14 drugs) comparison.

		k=1	2	3	4	5
	ndotj	174	549	815	3902	6041
Placebo	RR	1.0	1.0	1.0	0.7	0.6
	pvalue	0.99	0.98	0.99	0.99	0.99
Placebo+PPIs	RR	5.9	3.4	3.0	1.8	1.6
	pvalue	**0**	**0**	**0**	**0**	**0**
Ibandronate	RR	2.0	1.6	1.2	0.6	0.7
	pvalue	0	0	0.05	0.99	0.99
Ibandronate+PPIs	RR	1.8	1.6	1.6	0.9	1
	pvalue	0.50	0.23	0.24	0.99	0.99
Teriparatide	RR	0.1	0.1	0.1	0.1	0.1
	pvalue	0.99	0.99	0.99	0.99	0.99
Teriparatide+PPIs	RR		0.6	0.5	0.3	0.3
	pvalue		0.99	0.99	0.99	0.99
PTH	RR			3.9	1.5	1.7
	pvalue			**0**	**0**	**0**
PTH+PPIs	RR			5.9	2.0	2.3
	pvalue			**0**	**0**	**0**
Bazedoxifene	RR			1.7	0.7	0.5
	pvalue			0.99	0.99	0.99
Bazedoxifene+PPIs	RR				2.2	0.9
	pvalue				**0**	0.99
Lasoxifene	RR			0.4	1.6	1.8
	pvalue			0.99	**0**	**0**
Lasoxifene+PPIs	RR			1.1	1.9	2.0
	pvalue			0.99	**0**	**0**
Raloxifene	RR			4.0	0.9	0.6
	pvalue			0.46	0.99	0.99
Raloxifene+PPIs	RR			12.9	1.0	0.7
	pvalue			0.05	0.99	0.99

Some drugs are only available from k=3 period.

TABLE 6.7
(Conditional) Power and type-I error (type-I er) for simulation study.

						Performance of SeqLRT					
z	η	pr(1)	pr(2)	pr(3)	pr(4)	pr(5)	Power(1)	Power(2)	Power(3)	Power(4)	Power(5)
1	1.2	0.052	0.036	0.029	0.018	0.017	0.052	0.086	0.113	0.129	0.143
1	1.5	0.105	0.110	0.124	0.278	0.317	0.105	0.203	0.302	0.496	0.656
1	2.0	0.220	0.328	0.512	0.900	0.949	0.220	0.476	0.744	0.974	0.999
1	4.0	0.746	0.962	0.998	1.000	1.000	0.746	0.990	1.000	1.000	1.000
0.5	2.0	0.079	0.122	0.282	0.512	0.653	0.079	0.191	0.419	0.717	0.902
1	2.0	0.220	0.328	0.512	0.900	0.949	0.220	0.476	0.744	0.974	0.999
2	2.0	0.326	0.404	0.800	0.999	0.999	0.326	0.598	0.920	1.000	1.000
4	2.0	0.531	0.746	0.990	1.000	1.000	0.531	0.881	0.999	1.000	1.000
z	η	pr(1)	pr(2)	pr(3)	pr(4)	pr(5)	type-I er(1)	type-I er(2)	type-I er(3)	type-I er(4)	type-I er(5)
1	1.0	0.027	0.012	0.007	0.003	0.001	0.027	0.039	0.045	0.048	0.049
2	1.0	0.022	0.016	0.005	0.003	0.001	0.022	0.038	0.042	0.045	0.046
4	1.0	0.025	0.011	0.007	0.003	0.002	0.025	0.036	0.042	0.045	0.047
						Performance of LongLRT					
z	η	pr(1)	pr(2)	pr(3)	pr(4)	pr(5)			Unconditional powers		
1.0	1.2	0.036	0.019	0.021	0.025	0.045			NA		
1.0	1.5	0.087	0.083	0.130	0.412	0.583			NA		
1.0	2.0	0.197	0.298	0.580	0.981	0.997			NA		
1.0	4.0	0.760	0.973	1.000	1.000	1.000			NA		
0.5	2.0	0.129	0.174	0.299	0.711	0.881			NA		
1.0	2.0	0.197	0.298	0.580	0.981	0.997			NA		
2.0	2.0	0.381	0.501	0.896	1.000	1.000			NA		
4.0	2.0	0.601	0.893	0.997	1.000	1.000			NA		
z	η	pr(1)	pr(2)	pr(3)	pr(4)	pr(5)	cumer(1)	cumer(2)	cumer(3)	cumer(4)	cumer(5)
1.0	1.0	0.018	0.005	0.007	0.004	0.001	0.018	0.023	0.030	0.034	0.035
2.0	1.0	0.025	0.011	0.007	0.004	0.002	0.025	0.036	0.042	0.046	0.048
4.0	1.0	0.027	0.012	0.007	0.003	0.002	0.027	0.039	0.045	0.048	0.050

η has constant values 1, 1.2, 1.5, 2, 4 over looks. Pr(k) is the probability of rejecting the null hypothesis for kth study period (conditional power). Power(k) is the unconditional power of SeqLRT for kth study period. Cumer(k) is the cumulative error of LongLRT when data are simulated under the null hypothesis. NA: Not Applicable. $z = 1$ indicates that the sample size of the simulated data is equal to the sample size of the real data. $z = 0.5$ indicates that the sample size of the simulated data is equal to half of the sample size of the real data.

TABLE 6.8
(Conditional) Power and type-I error (type-I er) for simulation study.

Performance of SeqLRT										
	Look 1	Look 2	Look 3	Look 4	Look 5	Look 1	Look 2	Look 3	Look 4	Look 5
case	pr(1)	pr(2)	pr(3)	pr(4)	pr(5)	Power(1)	Power(2)	Power(3)	Power(4)	Power(5)
1	0.746	0.328	0.124	0.278	0.317	0.746	0.829	0.850	0.892	0.926
2	0.953	0.962	0.007	0.003	0.001	0.953	0.998	0.998	0.998	0.998
3	0.027	0.012	0.007	1.000	1.000	0.027	0.039	0.045	1.000	1.000
4	0.105	0.110	0.124	0.900	1.000	0.105	0.203	0.302	0.930	1.000
Performance of LongLRT										
	Look 1	Look 2	Look 3	Look 4	Look 5	Look 1	Look 2	Look 3	Look 4	Look 5
case	pr(1)	pr(2)	pr(3)	pr(4)	pr(5)	Unconditional powers				
1	0.760	0.298	0.177	0.412	0.583	NA				
2	0.962	0.973	0.009	0.004	0.001	NA				
3	0.018	0.005	0.009	1.000	1.000	NA				
4	0.087	0.083	0.177	0.981	1.000	NA				

η has different values over looks. For case 1: η is 4 for Look 1, 2 for Look 2, 1.5 for the remaining 3 looks; for case 2: η is 6 for Look 1, 4 for Look 2, and 1 for the remaining looks; for case 3: η is 1 for the first 3 looks and 4 for Look 4 and 6 for Look 5; for case 4: η is 1.5 for the first 3 looks, 2 for Look 4, and 4 for Look 5. z is 1 for all the cases in Table 6.8. Pr(k) is the probability of rejecting the null hypothesis for kth study period (conditional power). Power(k) is the unconditional power of SeqLRT for kth study period. NA: Not Applicable.

7

LRT-based Methodologies for Analysis of Multiple Studies

7.1 Background and Motivation

This chapter summarizes the LRT method for multiple studies, as proposed by Huang et. al. [82]. Meta-analysis approaches for multiple independent studies have become popular in medical research. In many observational and/or clinical trial studies, meta-analysis can be performed using either the study-level summary measures or patient-level information. For example, the studies can be integrated using a common statistical measure such as the study-level mean or effect size and computing a weighted average of this common measure using a statistical approach such as a fixed-effect model or a random-effects model [25]. The weights are usually related to the study-level sample sizes or within-study variation but may depend on other factors such as study quality, regions/countries, study time, study design (RCT or non-RCT), etc. This type of approach is referred to as the traditional meta-analysis and is extensively used to support evaluation of the efficacy and safety of drug products in pre- and post- approval process. The traditional meta-analysis of many large and small clinical trials, published studies, registries, and large clinical and/or observational databases, for thorough evaluation of clinical efficacy endpoints such as the mean change in the weight-loss or blood-pressure and hazard ratio in survival comparison, and clinical safety endpoints such as odds ratio, risk ratio, and absolute risk difference, has become a common practice for the modern-day pre- and post- market clinical/observational studies [25, 66]. For example, a number of meta-analyses of rosiglitazone trials for patients with type-2 diabetes have been conducted to evaluate the risk for myocardial infarction (MI) and cardiovascular mortality [113].

Using the traditional meta-analysis for safety evaluation, researchers can evaluate the point estimates and 95% confidence intervals for odds ratio or risk ratio of the drug-AE pair of interest from each study, combine the estimates through a fixed-effect model or a random-effects model, produce an overall estimate of the parameter of interest and its associated 95% confidence interval, and ultimately display the results using a forest plot.

Here, we intend to extend the traditional meta-analysis to safety signal detection, where relative risks (RRs) are commonly used when the drug exposure information is available, and are usually called the risk ratios. The relative event rates or proportional reporting rates are used in case of a lack of drug exposure information, which is usually the case in passive surveillance of medical products. It is important to explore safety signals in each study; however, when studying safety signals, researchers usually collect information from multiple trials (or studies) since a single clinical study with a focus on efficacy cannot provide sufficient information for safety events. The clinical studies, included in a large safety data or database, are usually independent studies with different protocols. A signal detected in one study may not be detected in other studies due to variation across studies (such as sample sizes, study sites, personnel, patients enrolled, study time, etc.).

Several methods have been developed for data mining or safety signal detection for exploring multiple drugs and AEs (e.g., proportional reporting ratios [45], reporting odds ratios [124], likelihood ratio tests [80, 81, 112], and Bayesian methods [22, 41, 74, 56]). However, these signal detection methods usually work on pooled large passive data and are not designed to incorporate the heterogeneity from multiple studies. Here, we present methods for drug safety signal detection (with an intent to control the type-I error and false discovery rate), for data with multiple studies, obtained from large observational databases such as FDA Event Reporting System (FAERS; https://open.fda.gov/data/faers/) or from clinical trial databases. The methods for multiple studies utilize the regular likelihood ratio test (LRT) for signal detection [80] and consist of a two-step approach for exploring safety signals from multiple studies/sources. In the first step, the basic LRT is applied to the safety data by study and in the second step, the basic LRT test statistics from different studies are combined to derive an overall test statistic for conducting the global test at a pre-specified level of significance. Overall, the data provides evidence of a signal if the global null is rejected in favor of the global alternative.

7.2 Methods

7.2.1 Summary of basic LRT with and without exposure information

As discussed in chapter 3, the maximum likelihood ratio (MLR) test statistic, for the one-sided alternative is

$$MLR = max_i(LR_{ij}I(\hat{p}_i > \hat{q}_i)) = max_i(\frac{n_{ij}}{E_{ij}})^{n_{ij}}(\frac{n_{.j} - n_{ij}}{n_{.j} - E_{ij}})^{n_{.j}-n_{ij}}I(\hat{p}_i > \hat{q}_i);$$

where the maximum is taken over $i = 1, \cdots, I$. Note that $E_{ij} = \frac{n_{i.}n_{.j}}{n_{..}}$ and $n_{..} = \sum_{i=1}^{I} n_{i.}$. Since logarithm $log(LR_{ij})$ is a monotonic (increasing) function of LR_{ij} , it is convenient to work with $MLLR = max_i(log(LR_{ij})I(\hat{p}_i > \hat{q}_i))$.

The above formulation was constructed assuming there is no drug exposure information in the large post-market safety database from passive surveillance system. In this case, the "no drug exposure" usually indicates that although we may know the number of AEs reported for a certain drug in a passive surveillance system, we may not know the number of patients who took the drug, or the drug exposure information for each person. Therefore, $n_{i.}$ is used to serve as an approximation of total drug use and relative reporting rates are compared for such an analysis using data from FDA adverse event reporting system (FAERS; https://open.fda.gov/data/faers/).

When the drug exposure for i^{th} drug (P_i) is available, all $n_{i.}$ can be replaced by P_i and the relative risks can then be compared with available drug exposure information (see some definitions in Huang et al. [81] and Chapter 6). Drug exposure information may be available in a legacy database including data from completed clinical trials, or data from ongoing clinical trials (for safety monitoring). In clinical trial data, the drug exposure for a patient is usually well-defined and pre-specified as the total dose taken by the patient during the study, or the exposure time from a certain dose of drug. However, in some cases, we may not have well-defined drug exposure information from completed clinical trials. For example, the precise drug exposure for the concomitant use of PPI is not collected in the studies included in Chapter 6, where we may have to impute the exposure with some reasonable assumptions.

Note that in order to detect signals using information from multiple studies, the drug exposure definition should be consistent and comparable across different studies in a single meta-analysis. Additional details are discussed in the applications.

In this case, the log likelihood ratio statistic is

$$log(LR_{ij}) = log[\frac{(\frac{n_{ij}}{P_i})^{n_{ij}}(\frac{n_{.j}-n_{ij}}{P_{.}-P_i})^{n_{.j}-n_{ij}}}{(\frac{n_{.j}}{P_{.}})^{n_{.j}}}] \tag{7.1}$$

$$= log[(\frac{n_{ij}}{E_{ij}})^{n_{ij}}] + log[(\frac{n_{.j}-n_{ij}}{n_{.j}-E_{ij}})^{n_{.j}-n_{ij}}] - log[(\frac{n_{.j}}{P_{.}})^{n_{.j}}]; i = 1, \cdots, I,$$

where $P_{.} = \sum_{i=1}^{I} P_i$, $\sum_{i=1}^{I} P_i/P_{.} = 1$, and $E_{ij} = \frac{P_i n_{.j}}{P_{.}}$.

Since the distribution of MLLR test statistic under the null hypothesis is not tractable, a Monte Carlo (MC) procedure is used to obtain the empirical distribution of MLLR by generating a large number of MC samples for the cell-report counts $(n_{1j}, \cdots, n_{Ij})$, for the jth AE, using Multinomial distribution $(n_{1j}, \cdots, n_{Ij})|n_{.j} \sim Mult(n_{.j}, (\frac{n_{1.}}{n_{..}}, \cdots, \frac{n_{I.}}{n_{..}}))$ with known $n_{.j}$ as the total number of events. If the drug exposure is available, the distribution is $(n_{1j}, \cdots, n_{Ij})|n_{.j} \sim Mult(n_{.j}, (\frac{P_1}{P_{.}}, \cdots, \frac{P_I}{P_{.}}))$. If the $MLLR$ based on the observed data, $MLLR_{data}$, is greater than the threshold value of $MLLR_{0.05}$(the upper 5th percentile point of the empirical distribution), the null hypothesis is rejected with alpha=0.05. The p-value of MLLR can be calculated as

$$1 - \frac{\text{rank of } MLLR_{data} \text{among } MLLR_{data} \text{and MLLRs from the empirical distribution}}{\text{1+total number of simulation for the empirical distribution generation}}.$$

The drug associated with $MLLR_{data}$ is then the most significant signal detected.

7.2.2 LRT analysis approaches for signal detection from multiple studies

Here, we present several LRT approaches based on the basic likelihood ratio test (LRT) for safety signal detection with multiple studies. Note that in the following, for each study s, $logLR_{ijs}$ or $logLR_{is}$ can be calculated using Equation 7.1.

Analysis of pooled data from several studies using basic LRT

For a total of S studies or datasets, $n_{ij}(= \sum_s n_{ijs})$ denotes the total of event/report counts for i^{th} drug and j^{th} AE, summed over all the S studies (note that here the subscript i is used for drug, and the row can be defined as either drug or AE depending on the interest). Using this definition of "pooled" n_{ij}, we can apply the basic LRT to detect the drug signals. However, the basic LRT applied to the pooled data may not control the type-I error as the MC simulation for obtaining the empirical distribution of the test statistic is carried out based on the pooled data, but not the study-level data, as seen in the simulation study.

Another issue with this analysis of pooled studies is that, it does not address the study to study variation (i.e., heterogeneity of studies). Study heterogeneity may stem from different sources including different study designs (prospective versus retrospective), endpoints, distributions of effect modifiers, or source of data. Therefore, analysis of the pooled studies without considering the heterogeneity may lead to biased results. This method is also vulnerable to Simpson's paradox [15, 139] and should be used with caution. For example, in a medical study for evaluating kidney stone treatment [30, 85], the paradoxical conclusion is that treatment A is more effective when used on patients with small stones, and also when used on patients with large stones, even though treatment B is more effective on all patients (combined data).

In the following subsections, two LRT approaches for incorporating study-level heterogeneity are presented.

Maximum of MLLR statistics from multiple studies (MMLLR)

For a total of S studies (with similar patients and objectives, and relevant for the purpose of current active/passive surveillance safety study), we define MLLR statistic for a fixed AE (j) of interest and s^{th} study as $MLLR_s = max_i(log(LR_{ijs})) = max_i(log(LR_{is}))$ dropping the suffix j. Thus, the test statistic for testing the global null hypothesis versus the global alternative hypothesis is the maximum of $MLLR_s$ over all studies defined by $MMLLR = max_s(MLLR_s)$. The empirical distribution of MMLLR can be obtained by Monte Carlo simulation by generating the null data with $n_{.s}$, P_{is} from observed data, the same relative risk for all rows from each study, $s = 1, ..., S$, and calculating $MMLLR = max_s(max_i(log(LR_{is}))$. Just as the basic LRT, MMLLR controls the type-I error.

A drug with MMLLR from observed data (for a particular study) is a signal if the related p-value (the rank of the MMLLR from the observed data among the MMLLR values obtained from empirical data divided by the total number of empirical data) is less than a pre-specified significance level (such as 0.05). Furthermore, if needed, we can identify secondary drug-study combinations as signals with logLR values $(log(LR_{is}), i = 1, \cdots, I, s = 1, \cdots, S)$ as the second largest, third largest, and fourth largest values among all values for the drug-study combinations.

Weighted LRT using Total Drug Exposure as Weight (wLRn)

In this subsection, we assume fixed j^{th} column and drop the suffix j in the following derivations.

Let P_{is} be the total drug exposure for i^{th} drug in s^{th} study. Then, the weighted log likelihood ratio, based on the total drug exposure, is defined as $wLR_i = \frac{\sum_{s=1}^{S_i} P_{is} log(LR_{is})}{\sum_{s=1}^{S_i} P_{is}}$, where S_i denotes the number of studies for the ith drug. Note that $S_i, i = 1, \cdots, I$ can be different for different rows, and wLR_i can be interpreted as the weighted average of logLR from different studies for ith row with weight P_{is}.

The test statistic for testing the global null hypothesis versus global alternative hypothesis is then defined as $MwLR = max_i(wLR_i)$, where the maximum is obtained over all drugs, $i = 1, \cdots, I$.

For statistical inference of wLRn method, the simulated null datasets are generated from a Multinomial distribution with $n_{.s}$ and P_{is} from observed data and with the same relative risk for all rows by study. The empirical distribution of wLR is formed by the 10,000 wLR_{sim} obtained from 10,000 simulated null data. The p-value of the wLR_{obs} is obtained by comparing the wLR_{obs} with the 10,000 wLR_{sim} values from the Monte Carlo process;

$$\text{p-value} = \frac{\#\text{of times } wLR_{\text{sim}} > wLR_{\text{obs}}}{10,000}.$$

If the wLR_{obs} for i^{th} drug (row) has p-value< 0.05, then the ith drug is a signal. After detecting the global signal, we can move to the 2nd largest, 3rd largest logLR or weighted logLR values, and so on for secondary signals.

The statistics discussed in Section 7.2.2 are summarized in Table 7.1.

7.3 Applications

We illustrate the use of the LRT methods by applying them to two datasets with multiple studies for safety signal exploration. The first dataset is hypothetical, but based on real PPI data from FDA legacy database. The second dataset includes 13 published clinical studies on Lipiodol (a contrast agent) as indicated by literature search. In both examples, we tried to include studies with similar features (such as similar patients, similar drugs, and similar objectives) for fair comparison.

7.3.1 Analysis of PPI data with two drugs and a composite AE

Proton Pump Inhibitors (PPIs) are a class of drugs that decrease gastric acid secretion through inhibition of the proton pump. PPIs are associated with increased risk of hip fractures (AE) [88, 145]. Huang et al. [81] (Chapter 6) evaluated whether the concomitant use of PPIs reduced the efficacy of test drugs intending to treat osteoporosis among targeted patients, using clinical trial data from FDA/OTS/OCS legacy database. This database contained data from 10 trials (including single arm studies, two-arm studies and three-arm studies). One medication (test drug for treating osteoporosis, active control, or placebo) was given to patients in one arm, and PPIs were given to patients in different arms concomitantly. The sample sizes of the trials range from hundreds to more than thousands. The main focus was on the composite AE (AEOST as defined in Chapter 6, Appendix 6.7.1), which includes many AE terms related to osteoporosis symptoms. After further examination of these data, we noticed that one trial did not have placebo arm, one trial had a placebo arm but did not have subjects with concomitant PPIs, and two trials did not have AEOST event reported in placebo+PPIs (PLandPPI) or placebo only (PL) groups. For illustration, we selected 6 trials with AEOST events reported and with partial subjects taking concomitant PPIs in the placebo arm. Note that the patients were randomized into test drug, active control, and placebo arms in those trials. The effect of PPIs and the other drugs (test drug and active control drugs) cannot be separated if they were used together in the test drug arm and active drug arm. Here, we illustrate the analysis of safety signals using the hypothetical data with 6 studies, which reflects the data pattern of the PPI clinical data for comparing PLandPPI and PL.

Two AEs considered here are the 1st occurrence of AEOST (denoted by 1occ) and repeated occurrences of AEOST (denoted by allocc). We evaluate the relative risks of the 1st occurrence of AEOST (or repeated occurrences of AEOST) for patients in PLandPPI group with exposure to placebo and concomitant PPIs vs. patients in PL group with exposure to placebo only. For 1occ analysis, n_{is} is the number of events for ith row (drug: placebo and PPIs together or placebo only) and s^{th} study with one event per subject (1st occurrence of the repeated AEOST); P_{is} is the exposure (sum of the exposure times in units of person-day) to the 1st occurrence of AEOST from all subjects) for i^{th} drug (row) and s^{th} study. For allocc analysis, n_{is} is the number of events for i^{th} drug (row) and s^{th} study when one subject has several repeated events for one AE such as AEOST; and P_{is} is the exposure (sum of the drug exposure time from all subjects) for i^{th} drug (row) and s^{th} study. Note that in this case, a subject's exposure time is defined as the time period of the subjects with placebo in PL group (time from taking placebo to the end of the study or drop-off). The exposure of concomitant PPIs in PLandPPI group is not well-recorded and is always shorter than placebo period. Therefore, we assume that the exposure of placebo and concomitant PPIs for subjects in PLandPPI group is the period of placebo exposure. The actual dose and exposure time of concomitant PPIs may vary by patient and the pattern may not be consistent with the total placebo exposure in the PLandPPI patients, which may introduce bias in evaluating the relative risk of PPIs together with placebo vs. placebo only.

Using traditional meta-analysis based on relative risks of safety issues, one may obtain an overall relative risk and 95% CI using fixed-effect or random-effects models (Borenstain et al. [25]). The τ^2 is 0 for the 1occ analysis and 0.07 for the allocc analysis. Therefore, the integrated results from fixed-effect model and random-effects model are almost the same. The overall relative risk and 95% CI is 1.87 (1.43, 2.45) for the 1occ analysis and 2.44 (2.02, 2.94) for the allocc analysis. The results are shown in a forest plot in Figure 7.1.

We also analyzed this data using the LRT methods namely simple pooled analysis with basic LRT, MMLR, and wLRn. Note that the application with two drugs can be easily extended to multiple drugs using the step-down procedure in LRT analysis methods (but not in traditional meta-analysis methods). For example, if one drug (Drug A) vs. other drugs is a signal, another drug (Drug B) can be a secondary signal if the value of the test statistic has a p-value smaller than 0.05 in case of more than two drugs.

The events and the relative risks (rr) of PLandPPI and PL with 95% CIs by study are summarized in Table 7.2. The results from basic LRT for individual study and the LRT analysis methods for multiple studies together are shown in Table 7.3. The 95% threshold in Table 7.3 is the 95th percentile of the empirical distribution of the related STAT.

Individual study analysis shows that the findings of the signals may vary in different studies with various levels of signal strength. The simple pooled analysis without considering the study variation, and the MMLR and wLRn methods each considering the study-level variability have consistent results (AEOST is a signal for PLandPPI group when compared with PL-only group). MMLR provides the strongest global signal of AEOST (along with the related study) as the integrated result. Stronger signal patterns were observed for the repeated occurrences analyses due to the large sample sizes. AEOST tends to be a signal for subjects taking concomitant PPIs (in PLandPPI group).

From MMLR method, the most significant global signal of AEOST (1st occurrence or repeated occurrences) in subjects taking concomitant PPIs (PLandPPI group) comes from the 2nd study (s=2). This signal for repeated occurrences is also seen in 4th study (s=4, with p-value 0.006), 5th study (s=5, with p-value 0.006), and 6th study (s=6, with p-value 0.009). The observed logLR for Studies 2, 4, 5, and 6 are all greater than the threshold of 2.47 for the analysis of repeated occurrences (allocc).

7.3.2 Analysis of lipiodol data with one drug and multiple AEs

Lipiodol (labeled Ethiodol in the USA), also known as ethiodized oil, is a poppyseed oil used by injection as a adiopaque contrast agent used to outline structures in radiological investigations [127, 18] such as in chemoembolization applications as a contrast agent in follow-up imaging [64].

In order to detect possible safety signals to document the safety of Lipiodol in selective intraarterial use for imaging liver lesions in adults with known hepatocellular carcinoma (HCC), thirteen studies (articles) were identified with maximum dose of Lipiodol as 15ml (as recommended in the drug label), from more than 100 articles included in NDA 09190/S-024 submission (https://www.accessdata.fda.gov/scripts/cder/drugsatfda/). The actual doses for different subjects varied. However, the maximum dose was reported to be 15ml for all subjects in the 13 studies selected. The subjects in these 13 studies were all adults (average age between 45 and 69, and average number between 11 and 257). All 13 articles were published between 1993 and 2009. A total of 27 AEs were reported in all the 13 studies for the drug under consideration (Lipiodol).

The number of subjects with a particular AE (n_{is}) is reported by study; note that one subject may have multiple AEs reported. Since the exact drug exposure time for each subject could not be determined from the articles, we assumed that the drug exposure is the same for each subject and considered it as one unit. The total drug exposure by study (P_{is}) is then the total number of subjects in each study, which in this case is the same for all rows ($P_{is} = P_s$).

Signals detected after applying the basic LRT to the individual study and the LRT methods to all the 13 studies (with a total of 27 AE terms) are shown in Tables 7.4 and 7.5. When the observed STAT (obsstat) is greater than the 95% threshold obtained from the empirical distribution under the null hypothesis of no signals, the related AE is a signal detected.

When interpreting the detected signals, one can consider lumping together similar AEs (with different AECODE codes) to form a group. For example, Post embolization syndrome (PES) (with the definition from http://radiopaedia.org/articles/post-embolisation-syndrome-1), including AECODE codes FEVER, VOMITTING, NAUSEA, and ABDOMINAL PAIN, is detected by all LRT analysis methods (Table 7.5).

The detected signals varied in the individual study analyses (Table 7.4). By simple pooled method and wLRn method, three AEs (all in PES group) were detected as signals with p-value less than 0.05 (Table 7.5). All the signals were integrated signals by considering the information from all the 13 studies.

Twenty one AE-study combinations were detected as signals by the MM-LLR method. PES was the most significant global signal detected among all the signals.

7.3.3 Summary of the two examples

We present the two examples (PPIs and Lipiodol) to demonstrate the performance of the proposed methods on two different types of datasets. Both examples use data from clinical trials with some exposure information. The AE signals detected can be designated as signals with higher relative risk. Because there is no exposure information and relative risk cannot be evaluated, similar applications can be conducted for data from passive surveillance system by evaluating reporting rates (see Ref. [80]). Without exposure information, the formula used in computing the likelihood ratios (Section 7.2.1) is different for different denominators.

The first example based on PPIs includes patients who were treated with multiple drugs over time (patients may have received different doses at different visits). In this example, the AE studied (AEOST) is an AE with many terms associated with osteoporosis. One could observe many repeated reports of the AEOST during the exposure duration. There are only two drug groups (drug groups as rows with $i = 1, 2$) and one selected composite AE (AEOST) for comparison. This is a simple case in signal detection and very similar to the set-up for traditional ways of data analysis in clinical trials. In this example, we compared the two drug groups with the fixed AE (AEOST).

In contrast, for the second example based on Lipiodol, contrast agents are used in discrete bursts and many patients have only a single exposure to the drug. Therefore, if the dose of the one-time injection is similar for each patient, we can assume that the drug exposure is the same for each subject and treat it as one unit. The P_i can then be imputed with number of patients without additional exposure information. In this example, there are 27 AEs (AEs as rows, $i = 1, \cdots, 27$) and one drug of interest. The purpose of signal detection is to identify the AEs with high relative risks by comparing one AE vs. other AEs for Lipiodol. There are a total of 27 comparisons (as opposed to 2 in the first example). The proposed LRT method can handle these multiple comparisons with false discovery rate (FDR) controlled [80].

7.4 Simulation

As discussed in Section 7.2.2, a simulation study is conducted to evaluate the performance of the LRT analysis methods, for data with multiple studies and available drug exposure information. The performance of traditional meta-analysis on risk ratio is also explored in simulated data with two rows.

7.4.1 Simulation setup

We simulated data using the information on the total number of studies, total number of rows, $n_{.s}$, and P_{is} from the datasets used in the illustration (see the cases in Table 7.6), equal relative risks for data generation under the global null hypothesis (without any safety signals by study) and with different relative risks associated with different rows (e.g., assigning the higher relative risk to the 1st row for data generation under the global alternative hypothesis). Note that each row corresponds to a drug or an AE. For example, a row corresponds to a drug in illustration 7.3.1 and to an AE in illustration 7.3.2.

For each study, if the relative risks are the same for different rows, the simulated null data are generated from the following Multinomial distribution (dropping suffix j),

$$(n_{1s}, \cdots, n_{Is})|n_{.s} \sim Mult(n_{.s}, (\frac{P_{1s}}{\sum_{i=1}^{I}(P_{is})}, \cdots, \frac{P_{Is}}{\sum_{i=1}^{I}(P_{is})})).$$

If the first row is a signal, with a higher relative risk, for each study, the simulated data (under global alternative) are generated from the following Multinomial distribution,

$$(n_{1s}, \cdots, n_{Is})|n_{.s} \sim Mult(n_{.s}, (\eta_{1s}\frac{P_{1s}}{\sum_{i=1}^{I}(\eta_{is}P_{is})}, \cdots, \eta_{Is}\frac{P_{Is}}{\sum_{i=1}^{I}(\eta_{is}P_{is})})),$$

where $\eta_{1s}\frac{P_{1s}}{\sum_{i}^{I}(\eta_{is}P_{is})} + \cdots + \eta_{Is}\frac{P_{Is}}{\sum_{i}(\eta_{is}P_{is})} = 1$. The relative risk of the first row vs. all other rows for s^{th} study with $\eta_{is} = 1, i = 2, \cdots, I$, is η_{1s}. The values of η_{1s} (same for different studies) in this simulation are selected to be 1, 1.2, 1.5, 2, and 3 (results with $\eta_{1s} = 1.2$ will not be shown in Table 7.6, but the powers are low in case of $\eta_{1s} = 1.2$). η values may also vary by study (for example, $\eta_{1s} = 1.5, 1.2, 3, 1, 1.3, 2$ for studies 1 to 6, respectively in the case with rr21 in Table 7.6).

The results for type-I error and power calculations, for different scenarios with equal relative risks (under global null) and different relative risks (under global alternative) are presented in Table 7.6. The drug exposure information P_i by row is obtained from the real data discussed in Section 7.3 (such as sim01occ, sim0allocc, and sim0lip). The drug exposure and case information are the same for scenarios sim01occ (null data) and sima1occ (alternative data), with only difference in the relative risks. The same rule was applied to all other null data and alternative data generation.

The total number of replications is 10,000 for the scenarios for type-I error evaluation and 1000 for the scenarios for power evaluation, respectively. The power is defined as the number of times the null hypothesis (no signal detected in each study) is rejected, divided by the total number of replications. When the data are generated with the assumption of no signals, the power becomes the type-I error.

7.4.2 Results

As shown in Table 7.6, the type-I error (or FDR) for data without any signals in each study stays low for wLRn and MMLR. The type-I error for the pooled method is slightly higher than the other methods with values up to 0.07 (not controlled). This is because the null data (counts) are generated from Multinomial distribution by study and then added over all studies. The pooled method is then applied to the pooled data (observed). The empirical distribution of statistics for decision-making are subsequently obtained by Monte Carlo procedure based on the pooled data, but not on the study-level data. The other two LRT analysis methods control the type-I error since both their statistics and empirical distributions are based on study-level data which are combined using different weighting approaches.

As shown in Table 7.6, the power is highest for pooled method, and moderate for wLRn and MMLR methods. The MMLR method is more conservative than wLRn. The power values increase with the increasing relative risk values assigned to the 1st row. Usually, for all methods, the power reaches 0.7–0.8 when the relative risk becomes 2 or 3. Since the sample size in scenario simaallocc is larger than the scenario sima1occ, the power values are higher for simaallocc scenarios with different relative risks. In the scenario with rr21 (with different η values by study), the pooled analysis no longer has the largest power.

Traditional meta-analysis (Borenstein et al. [25]) with test based on normal assumption (Z statistic) and the null hypothesis that the mean effect is 1 (relative risk case) or 0 (log of relative risk) is applied to several simulated data scenarios with two rows for power and type-I error evaluation. If the p-value (from the standard normal Z test) is less than 0.05, we reject the null hypothesis of relative risk (PLandPPI vs. PL) as 1. The type-I error is 0.067 and 0.070 for scenarios sim0allocc and sim01occ respectively. The results reflect the inflated error of the traditional meta-analysis for data with two rows (one comparison). With more than two rows (multiple comparison) in the data, we expect bigger type-I error from the traditional meta-analysis.

The power values of the traditional meta-analysis are 73%, 98%, and 100% for scenarios simaallocc with true relative risks for the 1st row as 1.5, 2, and 3, respectively. The powers for sima1occ scenarios are smaller than the simaallocc cases due to smaller sample size, but reasonably large for cases with relative risk 2 or above. The powers from the traditional meta-analysis are very low (about 5%) for the data generated with varying relative risks for different studies (scenarios simaallocc and sima1occ with rr21).

7.5 Discussion

In summary, we present the analysis using basic LRT on pooled data, MMLLR, and weighted LRT method (wLRn) identify signals for ith row (a drug or an AE) by incorporating the information from different studies. In addition, with MMLLR method, one can identify the global signal(s) for ith row (a drug or an AE) along with the studies containing that global signal(s). Multiple signals can be detected with step-down process embedded in LRT method for wLRn and MMLLR methods.

The traditional meta-analysis methods obtain a summary statistic based on the study-level statistics such as relative risk (also called risk ratio) by fixed-effect or random-effects models or other weighting methods. There are two steps in the traditional methods: first, obtaining the study-level statistic (odds ratio or risk ratio), and second, obtaining the summary statistic for overall evaluation using the study-level statistic. One may then use a normal approximation for the confidence interval construction and testing for statistical significance using the summary statistic. The two-step approach is also used by the proposed LRT methods as another way of exploring safety issues. However, in LRT methods (MMLLR and wLRn), the study-level statistics are logLR. Monte Carlo (MC) simulation is used for testing for significance of the summary statistic. The use of logLR and a step-down process for identifying secondary signals with smaller logLR values and the non-parametric MC simulation for empirical distribution of the logLR or summary of logLR using null datasets together, controls type-I error and FDR. In practice, one may consider conducting the traditional meta-analysis and the proposed signal detection method together in safety evaluation from multiple studies.

Normal distribution of the parameter estimates from different studies is commonly assumed in the fixed-effect model and random-effects model for traditional meta-analysis. Simulations have shown these methods to be relatively robust even under extreme violations of distributional assumptions in estimating heterogeneity [91] and calculating an overall effect size in traditional meta-analysis [90]. However, many meta-analyses include a small number of studies (such as 5) rendering the sample size inadequate to accurately estimate heterogeneity. In cases with limited studies, one can still use weighted LRT method using drug exposure as weight for safety signal exploration. Note that the weight can be study-sample-size or drug-exposure or can be defined by the researchers to reflect the importance of the different study-features. The proposed LRT methods are primarily appropriate for post-market safety evaluation with AE data collected from different studies (such as completed clinical trials or observational studies) and for safety signal monitoring using data from ongoing clinical trials.

When analyzing observational data from passive surveillance system such as FAERS, exposure information such as total number of subjects taking drugs, drug exposure time, or dose, is not available. Therefore, we can only evaluate reporting rate and the denominator for the reporting rate calculation is $n_{i.}$. When analyzing data from clinical trials, usually some information about exposure such as the number of patients, the dose for each patient, or the exposure time from taking drug to event, is available. Therefore, we can evaluate the risk with denominator P_i. When using the proposed method for combining information from multiple studies, one cannot combine information from observational data and clinical trial data. In a meta-analysis, we only apply the proposed method to studies with similar features, such as similar denominators, patient populations, study objectives, etc.

The proposed LRT methods output the p-values, which incorporate relative risk (rr) and exposure from different studies. For each study, an AE signal with higher rr and bigger exposure value may lead to a small p-value; and an AE with higher rr and small exposure value may not have a small p-value. The integrated AE signals with small p-values from all studies are affected by the combined information of the rr estimates and exposure information from all studies. Both relative risk and exposure by study are important pieces of information that can be included in the output in addition to the p-values from the proposed LRT method.

7.6 Tables and Figures

TABLE 7.1
Statistics in different methods (j is fixed and drop suffix j in the following formulation).

method	logLR or weighted logLR	Test-statistic (STAT)	most significant signal detected
pooled	$logLR_i$	$MLLR = max_i(log(LR_i))$	a row
MMLLR	$logLR_{is}$	$MMLLR = max_s max_i(log(LR_{is}))$	a row-study combination
wLRn	$wLR_i = \frac{\sum_{s=1}^{S_i} P_{is} logLR_{is}}{\sum_{s=1}^{S_i} P_{is}}$	$MwLR = max_i(wLR_i)$	a row

Either logLR or LR can be used. In addition to the most significant signal, secondary signals can also be identified.

TABLE 7.2
Summary of basic information of the PPIs study by trials.

Study	PL N(subject)	PL event	PL exposure (person-day)	PLandPPI N(subject)	PLandPPI event	PLandPPI exposure (person-day)	rr (95% CI)
1st occurrence of AEOST analyses							
s=1	309	14	168947	25	1	10225	1.18(0.16, 8.97)
s=2	1647	77	1534190	245	20	181753	2.19(1.34, 3.58)
s=3	210	11	133813	20	2	9822	2.48(0.55, 11.17)
s=4	1058	167	470833	165	30	56845	1.49(1.01, 2.19)
s=5	950	144	713856	32	8	19575	2.03(0.99, 4.13)
s=6	150	17	87481	9	3	2884	5.35(1.57, 18.26)
all s	4324	430	3109120	496	64	281104	1.65(1.27, 2.14)
Repeated occurrences of AEOST analyses							
s=1	309	30	173796	25	4	10383	2.23(0.78, 6.33)
s=2	1647	179	1575058	245	67	196698	3.00(2.26, 3.97)
s=3	210	13	136128	20	3	10381	3.03(0.86, 10.62)
s=4	1058	228	513109	165	48	64764	1.67(1.22, 2.28)
s=5	950	169	789274	32	14	24188	2.70(1.57, 4.66)
s=6	150	21	95959	9	5	4266	5.36(2.02, 14.20)
all s	4324	640	3283324	496	141	310680	2.33(1.94, 2.79)

rr is the relative risk for PLandPPI vs. PL.

TABLE 7.3
Results of PPIs data (for PLandPPI vs. PL).

	1st occurrence of AEOST			repeated occurrences of AEOST		
	obsstat	pvalue	95% threshold	obsstat	pvalue	95% threshold
individual study analysis using basic LRT						
s=1	0.12	0.99	1.79	0.93	0.438	1.96
s=2	4.16	0.004	2.10	24.28	0	2.00
s=3	0.56	0.61	1.73	1.18	0.243	1.18
s=4	1.83	0.07	2.04	4.63	0.006	2.03
s=5	1.54	0.137	1.69	4.88	0.006	2.27
s=6	2.43	0.031	0.97	3.97	0.009	1.17
simple pooled analysis using basic LRT						
	6.12	0.003	1.78	34.27	0.0	1.83
MMILR						
	4.16	0.006 (from s=2)	2.43	24.28	0 (from s=2)	2.47
wLRn						
	2.81	0.019	1.92	14.02	0	2.12

obsstat is the statistics shown in Table 7.1 for different methods, obtained from the observed data.

TABLE 7.4
Analysis of Lipiodol data (individual study analysis).

Studies	# signals	AE terms	obsstat	pvalue	95% threshold
s=1	0	None			3.33
s=2	4	**ABDOMINAL PAIN**	171.8	0	3.93
		FEVER	157.5	0	
		ANOREXIA/LOSS OF APPETITE	130.4	0	
		VOMITTING	11.6	0	
s=3	3	**FEVER**	192.9	0	4.50
		ABDOMINAL PAIN	56.7	0	
		NAUSEA	8.5	0	
s=4	2	**FEVER**	7.8	0	4.77
		ABDOMINAL PAIN	4.8	0.003	
s=5	3	**FEVER**	29.4	0	4.72
		ABDOMINAL PAIN	6.7	0	
		NAUSEA	4.73	0.007	
s=6	1	**POST EMBOLIZATION SYNDROME**	29.6	0	3.73
s=7	1	SHOULDER PAIN	32.2	0	4.89
s=8	2	**VOMITTING**	23.6	0	4.89
		ABDOMINAL PAIN	7.3	0	
s=9	4	HEMATOLOGICAL or BONE MARROW TOXICITY	34.1	0	4.02
		FEVER	9.3	0	
		BILIRUBIN RELATED ABNORMALITIES	4.7	0.015	
		HEPATIC PEDICULITIS	4.7	0.015	
s=10	3	PAIN NOS	26.8	0	3.47
		FEVER	24.1	0	
		VOMITTING	16.7	0	
s=11	2	**FEVER**	121.8	0	3.73
		PLUERAL EFFUSION	15.5	0	
s=12	1	**FEVER**	4.5	0.008	4.38
s=13	1	RESPPIRATORY DISTURBANCE	3.3	0	3.18

Bold AE terms are in PES group.

TABLE 7.5
Analysis of Lipiodol data from multiple studies (integrated results over studies).

Analysis	# signals	AE term (obsstat)	95% threshold
simple pooled analysis	4	**FEVER** (473.6) **ABDOMINAL PAIN** (195.2) ANOREXIA/LOSS OF APPETITE (61.0) **VOMITTING** (10.7)	3.93
wLRn	4	**FEVER** (89.7), **ABDOMINAL PAIN** (66.8) ANOREXIA/LOSS OF APPETITE (44.0) **VOMITTING** (5.9)	1.56
MMLLR	21[a]	**FEVER** (192.9), **ABDOMINAL PAIN** (171.8) ANOREXIA/LOSS OF APPETITE (130.4) HEMATOLOGICAL/BONE MARROW TOXICITY (34.1) SHOULDER PAIN (32.2) **POST EMBOLIZATION SYNDROME** (29.6) PAIN NOS(30.0), VOMITTING (26.8) PLUERAL EFFUSION (18.2), **NAUSEA** (8.5)	6.40

[a] note that 21 AE-study combination signals are detected by MMLR method, p-value is 0 for the most significant one (for AE FEVER and 3rd study (s=3)). 10 AE terms were reported in those signals ignoring the study information and are shown in the column for AE term with maximum observed logLR over the studies.

TABLE 7.6
Type-I error (or FDR) for cases with data generated under null hypothesis (all relative risks as 1) and power (%) for cases with data generated under alternative hypothesis (varying relative risks).

cases	description	LRT Methods		
		pooled	wLRn	MMLLR
type-I error				
sim0allocc	with p_{is} and $n_{.s}$ from real data allocc case in Table 2, rr1	0.055	0.047	0.050
sim01occ	with p_{is} and $n_{.s}$ from real data 1st occurrence case in Table 2, rr1	0.073	0.047	0.049
sim0LIP	with p_{is} and $n_{.s}$ from real Lipiodol data, 13 studies, 27 rows, rr1	0.046	0.045	0.038
Power				
simaallocc	rr2	86.7	67.2	48.9
simaallocc	rr3	99.3	98.4	92.8
simaallocc	rr4	100	100	99.9
sima1occ	rr2	74.3	37.2	30.1
sima1occ	rr3	97.5	77.0	66.5
sima1occ	rr4	100	98.2	96.9
simaLIP	rr2	38.3	23.4	11.1
simaLIP	rr3	95.0	86.3	63.0
simaLIP	rr4	100	100	99.3
simaallocc	rr21	32.9	100	99.9
sima1occ	rr21	16.7	11.5	8.0

rr1, rr2, rr3, and rr4 are for cases with the 1st row with relative risk (η_1) as 1, 1.5, 2, and 3, respectively (all other rows have relative risk as 1). In rr1, rr2, rr3, and rr4 cases, η_1 is the same for all 6 studies. In rr21 case: $\eta_1 = 1.5, 1.2, 3, 1, 1.3, 2$, for 1st row in studies 1 to 6, respectively.
For case sim01occ, $n_{1s}(= 1, 20, 2, 30, 8, 3)$ are the counts of the 1st AEOSET events for PLandPPI group from studies 1 to 6, respectively. $P_{1s}(= 10225, 181753, 9822, 56845, 19575, 2884)$ are the exposure for PLandPPI group from studies 1 to 6, respectively. $n_{2s}(= 14, 77, 11, 167, 144, 17\ )$ are the counts of 1st AEOSET events for PL group from studies 1 to 6, respectively. $P_{2s}(= 168947, 1534190, 133813, 470833, 713856, 87481)$ are the exposure for PL group from studies 1 to 6, respectively.
The n_{is} and $P_{is}, i = 1, 2$ for case sim0allocc can also be found in Table 2 (for repeated occurrences of AEOST).
For case sim0LIP, the n_{is} and $P_{is}(i = 1, \cdots, 27$ and $s = 1, \cdots, 13)$ cannot be listed here due to space limitation. The values of n_{is} range from 0 to 128, and the values of $P_{is} = P_s$ range from 11 to 257.

FIGURE 7.1
Forest plot of relative risk and 95% CI by study and summary (integrated using fixed effect model) relative risk using traditional meta-analysis methods (1occ analysis (on the left) and allocc analysis (on the right)).

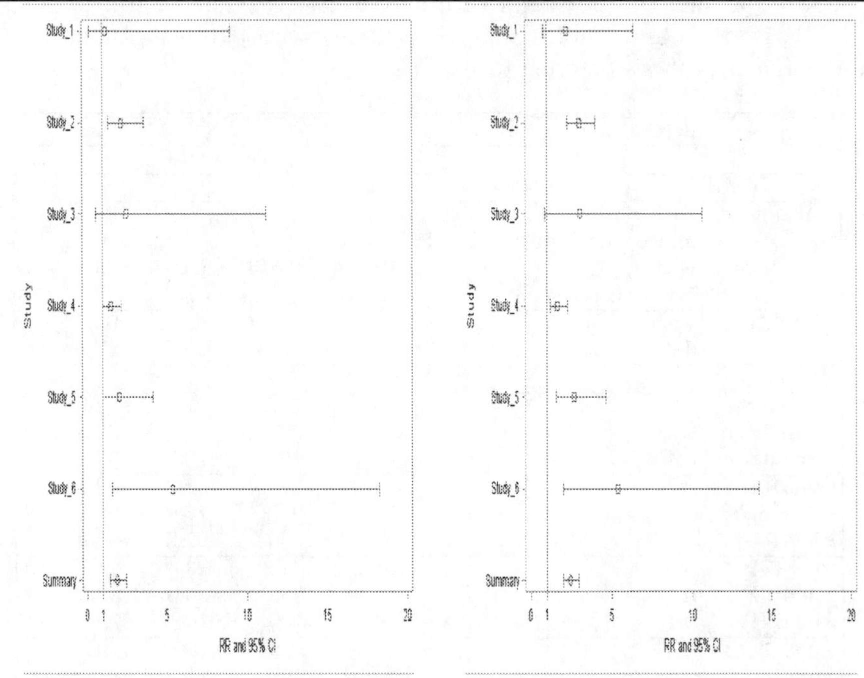

Part III

Additional Frameworks

8

LRT Methods in Medical Device Safety Evaluation

8.1 Background

The United States (US) medical device industry plays an important role in the medical care of patients world-wide. The safety, effectiveness, and security of medical devices in United States is monitored by the U.S. Food and Drug Administration (FDA). The 21st Century Cures Act, enacted in December 2016, authorized FDA to modernize its regulatory framework and make its review process more efficient [58]. With a focus on the total product life cycle, FDA is streamlining its science-based and patient-centered regulatory approach toward medical devices to foster medical device innovation and allow patients timely access to high quality, safe, and effective medical devices [59]. With a record number of approved and cleared devices, FDA is enhancing its pre- and post-market safety tools, including the establishment of a new pre- and post-market National Evaluation System for health Technology (NEST).

Medical Device Reporting (MDR) is one of the post-market surveillance systems that FDA uses to monitor device performance, detect potential device-related safety-issues, and contribute to benefit-risk assessments of these products [107]. However, with thousands of new devices being marketed over past several decades, conducting monitoring and surveillance of the medical devices without the help of automatic analytical tools becomes challenging. Recent high-profile failures of new devices also raised concerns about the current safety monitoring system for medical devices. One such example is textured breast implants, which were found to be associated with a rare cancer [60] and were recalled by FDA in July, 2019. Another example is paclitaxel-coated balloons and stents, which were linked to a possible increased risk of death at two years and beyond in patients with peripheral artery disease (PAD) [87]. The need to create a robust system for medical device safety monitoring is pressing. However, unlike the well-established drug safety surveillance system developed and utilized within FDA, the device safety surveillance system is still at an early stage of development due to multiple factors, including lack of data standardization in existing databases, lack of analytical tools, etc.

Adverse events (AEs) associated with the use of medical devices can have serious consequences, including life-threatening injuries and death. However, monitoring device safety and identifying safety signals can be challenging due to factors related to both the device and patient. For instance, medical devices can be comprised of multiple complex parts, have several indications for use, and can be used off-label [143].

The HeartWare Ventricular Assist Device (HVAD) is an example of one such complex device with different indications for use in subjects with multiple comorbidities. In 2017, HVAD approval was expanded to include destination therapy (DT) in addition to its original approval for bridge-to-transplant therapy (BTT) [134]. The HVAD and the HeartMate II are commonly implanted left ventricular assist devices (LVADs) worldwide and in addition to the HeartMate III, the only LVADs currently on the U.S. market with FDA approval for both BTT and DT ([39, 109, 110]). HeartMate III is not examined in the following example due to limitations of the data source. Given the critical health burden of heart failure and the limited availability of cardiac transplants, there has been a rapid growth in the use of LVADs ([122, 126]). This in turn has presented a need for timely post-market surveillance to evaluate their safety and effectiveness, as well as to monitor and reduce the occurrence of AEs [71].

In Sections 8.2 and 8.3, the basic LRT method and modified LRT method are illustrated for the LVAD safety evaluation using post-market MDR data (Section 8.2, [144]) and clinical trial safety data (Section 8.3, [86]). In Section 8.4, the spatial LRT method ([75]) is used to explore the spatial-cluster signals of the LVADs for an AE of interest (stroke) using simulated data.

Post-market may contain data from many studies, regions, or registries. In Section 8.5, the modified LRT method (discussed in Chapter 7) is applied to the safety data with multiple studies for exploring mortality safety signal associated with paclitaxel-coated products (device) in treating patients with peripheral arterial disease.

8.2 LRT Methods for Device Data from MDR

In this section, the LRT-based method is applied to identify AE signals associated with LVADs using MDR data. In addition, the PRR and two Bayesian methods (sB and BCPNN) are also used for comparison.

8.2.1 MDR data for LVADs

Each year, nearly one million medical devices-related AEs such as death, serious injuries, or device malfunctions are reported to FDA through the MDR system [63]. The coding system for outcomes in the MDR system is based on the International Medical Device Regulators Forum (IMDRF) documents. As part of mandatory reporting, manufacturers input patient and device codes directly into the MDR system. Given the considerable number of reports, a major challenge in analyzing MDR data is to extract the relevant information (i.e., patient AEs and device problems) from the narratives. More details about MDR data can be found in Chapter 1.

Compared to the number of reports in the FDA Adverse Event Reporting System (FAERS) for drugs, that in the MDR system is much smaller. Each unique report contains multiple entries and each entry represents a patient AE or device malfunction (device problem code). Patient AEs include deaths as well as injuries that are life-threatening, result in disability, or physical harm, or require medical intervention or hospitalization [12]. Device problems include issues related to device functionality, user facilities, user interaction, and physical properties [12] and are of concern given that they can potentially lead to patient AEs. LVADs in the MDR data have been found to be one of the device classes with high AE rates for both patient AEs and device problems. Therefore, in the following sections, we explore LVAD safety data from the MDR system.

8.2.2 Exploration of the device data

AE signals detected by LRT method

The LRT method is employed to detect AE signals or AEs that have a significantly higher relative reporting rate than other AEs for HeartMate II. After investigating a total of 110,927 AE entries from 2007 to 2019, 22 patient AE terms are detected as safety signals from a total of 310 patient AE terms using the LRT method with a criterion of p-value < 0.05.

Tour patient AE terms coded as "No Information", "Test Result", "No Code Available", and "Not Applicable" are not appropriately defined. Table 8.1 shows the remaining 18 significant AE signals detected by the LRT method after removing these four. Thrombosis, an important safety risk reported with this type of device [131], is also detected as a signal by the LRT method (Table 8.1).

AE signals detected by other methods

In addition to the LRT method, AEs for LVADs are analyzed using other contemporary statistical AE signal detection methods including two Bayesian methods (BCPNN and sB), as well as the traditional Frequentist PRR method. With the pre-specified signal detection criteria noted in Table 8.2, we detected 29 signals by BCPNN, 36 by sB, and 108 by PRR. Due to the limitation of space, Table 8.2 only lists 29 signals detected by BCPNN along with their corresponding sB and PRR results. Overall, the LRT method is the most conservative method as it controls for false positive signals as compared to the other evaluated methods when examining the total number of detected signals.

The AE signals detected by these methods are illustrated in a Venn diagram (Figure 8.1) and compared against each other. The diagram shows that all the signals detected by the LRT method are confirmed by the other methods. The signals detected by BCPNN are a subset of the signals identified by sB. The AE signals detected by any of the three methods (BCPNN, sB or LRT) are also detected by PRR.

AE signals over time using the LRT method

To understand the trends and to monitor AE signals over time for HeartMate II, we extracted AE data from year 2007 to 2019 and applied the longitudinal-LRT method to analyze them cumulatively by year [81]. The longitudinal-LRT uses a monotone alpha-spending function that distributes the total amount of allocated type-I error (alpha) of 0.05 over different yearly-looks to ensure the control of type-I error at each look and also for all looks. This method detects AE signals at each year using the specified value of alpha for that year (details are discussed in Section 6.3).

For illustration, Figure 8.2 shows the five most frequently observed AEs and their logarithm values of likelihood ratio (i.e., LogLR, a relative measure of the magnitude of the signal using the LRT method) over years from 2007 to 2019. Dark dots represent the AE signals detected by the longitudinal-LRT method. If an AE is detected as a signal at a particular look and continues to be a signal at several other looks, the signal has a higher chance of being a real safety concern. We noticed that AE signals such as thrombosis started since 2010, hemolysis since 2012, infection since 2014, hematuria since 2014, and death since 2013.

AE term and SOC signals

From the links https://www.fda.gov/medical-devices/mdr-adverse-event-codes/coding-resources and https://tools.meddra.org/wbb/, one can identify whether an AE in the MDR data is a lower level term (LLT), a preferred term (PT), or neither. Once a LLT/PT term is identified, the higher level terms defined in MedDRA (such as system organ class (SOC)) can also be identified in the MDR data. Some AE terms in MDR data may not be LLT/PT terms defined in MedDRA.

The modified LRT method (discussed in Section 4.3) can be used to detect safety signals in the data with two layers (a layer with AE terms that could be LLT/PT terms, and a layer with SOC terms). In the current example, only two SOCs are considered and the results are shown in Table 8.3. In addition to the AE signals, two SOCs ("Blood and Lymphatic System Disorders" and "Cardiac Disorders") are detected as signals in this MDR data.

AE signals using device problem code

In addition to patient problem codes, MDR data also has device problem codes (further details are discussed in chapter 1). Table 8.4 shows the safety signals for HeartMate II, as detected by the LRT method when examining device problem codes in MDR data. The signals include device stops intermittently, infusion, break, electrical shorting, and others.

8.2.3 Remarks

In the HeartMate II example, thrombosis has been identified as a signal since 2010. In 2013, researchers at the Cleveland Clinic published a report for the unexpected abrupt increase in LVAD thrombosis [134]. Their findings indicate that the increasing rate of pump thrombosis related to the use of HeartMate II is associated with substantial morbidity and mortality. Using the LRT method, we notice that thrombosis is an AE signal among all other AEs for HeartMate II starting in 2010 and continues to be a signal in subsequent years.

The FDA issued a safety communication in 2015 [49] regarding serious adverse events related to LVADs, which included increased rate of pump thrombosis and bleeding complications related to the pump for HeartMate II. Early identification of an AE signal can help clinicians better determine the most appropriate treatment plan for individual patients. This example shows that the LRT method can be used in the early detection of AE signals and that post-market data collection and analyses are important after the approval of a device.

8.3 Safety Evaluation in Treatment vs. Control Group for Medical Device

In the previous section, the basic LRT method was applied to identify AE signals for LVADs from MDR data. The current section presents the modified LRT and conventional z-test methods with exposure information for comparing safety signals between two devices in the presence of multiple AEs using clinical trial data.

8.3.1 Data source

Data are obtained from a previous study by Rogers et al. [123], which aimed to assess the safety and effectiveness of HeartWare relative to HeartMate II as destination therapy (DT) among subjects with chronic, advanced left ventricular failure in a multicenter randomized clinical trial. The data from the "as-treated population" included: 296 subjects implanted with the HeartWare LVAD and 149 others implanted with the HeartMate II device. The analysis is performed on the 26 AEs that are reported up to two-years post-implant by Rogers et al. These AEs and AE definitions are the same as those defined and captured in the Interagency Registry for Mechanically Assisted Circulatory Support (INTERMACS) and are clinically important for the safety and effectiveness of LVAD. While survival free of disabling stroke or device removal due to malfunction or failure is an appropriate primary endpoint for the original Rogers et al. study, the focus of this modified LRT methodology is identifying potential signals among many reported AEs. Components of the primary endpoint (stroke, death, and pump replacement) are all considered as separate AEs in the following analysis.

8.3.2 Statistical models

Two statistical methods, the modified LRT method and the Z-test with p-values adjusted by the Benjamini-Hochberg (BH) procedure [23], are utilized to analyze data on 26 AEs presented in Roger et. al. [123], Tables 3 and S13. The number of subjects with AE_i are represented by n_{iT} and n_{iC}, where i represents the ith AE, T represents HeartWare (i.e., treatment group), and C represents HeartMate II (i.e., control group). It is assumed that n_{iT} and n_{iC} follow independent Poisson distributions with means $\lambda_{iT}P_T$ and $\lambda_{iC}P_C$, respectively, where P_T and P_C are the total known exposure-time of all subjects in the two groups, and λ_{iT} and λ_{iC} are unknown parameters denoting the risk for the ith AE during the total exposure-time for the two groups, respectively. For each AE_i, the model and maximum likelihood estimates (MLEs) of parameters are shown below:

Model:

$$n_{iT} \sim Pois(P_T\lambda_{iT}); n_{iC} \sim Pois(P_C\lambda_{iC}); n_{iT} \perp n_{iC}$$
$$H_{0i} : \lambda_{iT} = \lambda_{iC} = \lambda_i \; vs. \; H_{ai} : \lambda_{iT} > \lambda_{iC}$$

MLEs under H_{ai} are $\hat{\lambda}_{iT} = \frac{n_{iT}}{P_T}; \hat{\lambda}_{iC} = \frac{n_{iC}}{P_C}; i = 1, \cdots, I$. MLEs under H_{0i} are $\hat{\lambda}_i = \frac{n_{iT}+n_{iC}}{P_T+P_C}, i = 1, \cdots, I$.

Based on the above model, two statistical methods for safety signal identification are examined: the conventional z-test with p-value adjustment and the modified LRT.

8.3.3 Conventional Z-test with P-value adjustment

The conventional Z-test is derived to analyze individual AEs using normal approximation:

$$\frac{\hat{\lambda}_{iT} - \hat{\lambda}_{iC}}{\sqrt{var(\hat{\lambda}_{iT} - \hat{\lambda}_{iC})_{H_{0i}}}} \sim Z(0,1)$$

$$var(\hat{\lambda}_{iC}) = \frac{\hat{\lambda}_{iC}}{P_C}; var(\hat{\lambda}_{iT}) = \frac{\hat{\lambda}_{iT}}{P_T}; var(\hat{\lambda}_{iT} - \hat{\lambda}_{iC})_{H_{0i}} = (\frac{1}{P_T} + \frac{1}{P_C})\hat{\lambda}_i.$$

$$\text{P-value for} AE_i = p(Z > \frac{\hat{\lambda}_{iT} - \hat{\lambda}_{iC}}{\sqrt{var(\hat{\lambda}_{iT} - \hat{\lambda}_{iC})_{H_{0i}}}}).$$

For each individual AE_i, the hypothesis is $H_{0i} : \lambda_{iT} = \lambda_{iC} = \lambda_i$ versus $H_{ai} : \lambda_{iT} > \lambda_{iC}$; thus, the one-sided test is performed to assess whether the risk for AE_i in the treatment group is larger than that in the control group. Considering that multiple AEs (I=26) are analyzed separately, and multiple statistical tests are performed, multiplicity adjustment is needed. Here, the BH procedure is applied to adjust the raw p-values to control for FDRs.

8.3.4 Modified LRT

Instead of conducting tests for multiple AEs separately one by one using Z-tests, the basic LRT-based approach (discussed in Chapter 3) is modified to perform tests for multiple AEs simultaneously. Using the Poisson model described above, the log likelihood ratios (LLR_i) for each AE_i for a one-sided test is first computed:

$$LLR_i = \frac{L_{H_a}}{L_{H_0}} = log\left(\frac{(\hat{\lambda}_{iC})^{n_{iC}}(\hat{\lambda}_{iT})^{n_{iT}}}{(\hat{\lambda}_i)^{n_{iC}+n_{iT}}}\right)I(\hat{\lambda}_{iT} > \hat{\lambda}_{iC}),$$

where $I(A)$ denotes the indicator of set A.

LLR_i can be written as

$$LLR_i = log((\frac{n_{iC}}{E_{iC}})^{n_{iC}} \times (\frac{n_{iT}}{E_{iT}})^{n_{iT}})I(\hat{\lambda}_{iT} > \hat{\lambda}_{iC}),$$

where $E_{iC} = (n_{iC} + n_{iT})(\frac{P_C}{P_T+P_C})$; $E_{iT} = (n_{iC} + n_{iT})\frac{P_T}{P_T+P_C}$ are the expected counts in the control and treatment arms under H_{0i}.

Then

$$LLR_i = log((\frac{n_{iC}/(n_{iC}+n_{iT})}{P_C/(P_T+P_C)})^{n_{iC}} \times (\frac{n_{iT}/(n_{iC}+n_{iT})}{P_T/(P_T+P_C)})^{n_{iT}})I(\frac{n_{iT}}{n_{iC}} > \frac{P_T}{P_C}), \tag{8.1}$$

Instead of testing multiple null hypotheses for each individual AE_i, the modified LRT method tests the global null hypothesis $H_0 : \cap_{i=1}^{I} H_{0i}$ versus the global alternative hypothesis $H_a : \cup_{i=1}^{I} H_{ai}$, with a global test statistic $MLLR = max_i(LLR_i)$. To perform this test, a Monte Carlo (MC) simulation is adopted to find the empirical distribution of $MLLR = max_i(LLR_i)$, under the null hypothesis (H_0). Under the null hypothesis, for each simulation m, the number of subjects with AE_i for the treatment and control groups are simulated by

$$(n_{iT}^{(m)}, n_{iC}^{(m)})|n_i \sim Multinomial(n_i; (\frac{P_T}{P_T+P_C}, \frac{P_C}{(P_T+P_C)}));$$

$m = 1, \cdots, M(= 1000); i = 1, 2, \cdots, I$ where $n_i = n_{iT} + n_{iC}$. The MC simulation is conditional on the sum, $n_{iT} + n_{iC}$, for each row (AE). The p-value for each AE_i is determined by ranking each observed LLR_i in the empirical distribution of $MLLR(p_i = \frac{\sum_{m=1}^{M} I(MLLR^{(m)} \geq LLR_i)}{M})$ and AEs with p-values less than 0.05 are identified as safety signals. Specifically, the LLR values from the observed data (ordered from largest to smallest) are compared with the maximum of $MLLR$ from simulated null data assuming that $\hat{\lambda}_{iC} = \hat{\lambda}_{iT}$ for all the AEs ($i = 1, \cdots, I$).

If the observed MLLR for a given row is larger than the threshold computed from the MC simulation, then the row associated with the MLLR is identified as a safety signal. The consecutive rows are then evaluated (i.e., first row to the 2nd row, 3rd row, etc.) until the LLR for a row is smaller than the threshold. The modified LRT controls for the overall type-I error and FDR through this maximization process, i.e., $MLLR = max(LLR_i)$ and stepwise approach.

8.3.5 Results

Results with LRT on single layer (AE terms)

Table 8.7 represents the results from both the modified LRT test and Z-test with BH procedure. In this dataset, the exposure-times (P_T and P_C), as measured in person-years, are the sum of years that participants are at risk for experiencing an AE. Overall, 410 patient-years are evaluated for the HeartWare LVAD (HVAD) group, and 204 subjects-years are evaluated for the HeartMate II group [123]. Both the modified LRT method and Z-test with BH procedure indicate that subjects utilizing HVAD have greater incident stroke than those using HeartMate II (p-values for analysis with time at risk: p=0.002 for LRT and p=0.005 for the Z-test with BH). A potential safety signal can further be quantified and assessed using the incidence rates by device and rate ratio. The incidence rate of stroke for HVAD subjects is 21.5 cases per 100 person-years ($88/410 \times 100$), while that for HeartMate II subjects is 8.8 cases per 100 person-years ($18/204 \times 100$). The rate ratio for stroke when comparing HVAD to HeartMate II subjects is 2.44 (0.215/0.088) with a 95% confidence interval ranging from 1.46 to 4.04, indicating that HVAD subjects have 2.44 times the rate of stroke as compared to HeartMate II subjects. For illustrative purpose of the method, it is assumed that exposure information is not available and every patient is treated with the same unit of time of exposure, so that the total exposure (P_T and P_C) is the sum of the total number of subjects. Both statistical tests also identify stroke as a safety signal for HVAD subjects as compared to HeartMate II subjects (p-values for analysis without time at risk: p=0.025 for LRT and p=0.027 for the Z-test with BH). Although the overall results are similar with and without time at risk included in the analysis, some p-values are smaller when person-years are considered. For wound dehiscence, the p-values for the Z-test with BH are not applicable due to there being zero subjects for both devices.

Results from LRT on double layers: AE terms and SOCs

The above analysis focused on identifying signals as AE term when comparing two groups (such as treatment vs. control). In this illustration, the AE terms are used as defined in Roger et al. [123]. In practice, one may also be interested in signals as combined AE terms or SOC including multiple AE terms. For example, bleeding events, hemolysis, and thrombocytopenia can be categorized into the SOC of blood and lymphatic system disorders; right heart failure, aortic valve incompetence, cardiac arrhythmia, cardiac tamponade, and myocardial infarction can be categorized into the SOC of cardiac disorders.

Using the idea from the modified LRT discussed in Section 4.3, we may consider subset index, g, to be AE terms plus any combinations of AE terms within the two SOCs (blood and lymphatic system disorders and cardiac disorders). In practice, one may add more SOCs for the analysis. The LLR values using Equation 8.1 are calculated for the g. In Table 8.8, we define g as the AE terms plus the two SOCs including all AE terms within a SOC for illustration. Stroke is still the only detected signal and there are two additional rows for the two SOCs with related counts and p-values.

8.3.6 Performance evaluation using simulation

An important consideration is detecting signals from a rare AE, which can be challenging in post-market safety surveillance. The small number of events usually limits the power of safety signal detection methods to claim statistical significance. Results from simulations conducted to evaluate the effect of sample size, including rare events, on the performance of the modified LRT method and the Z-test with BH adjustment, are included in this section.

In the simulation, data are generated using marginal count data and the exposure information obtained from the Rogers et al. [123] study to capture the observed data patterns.

Simulation model:

Suppose $n_{iT} \sim Pois(P_T \lambda_{iT}); n_{ic} \sim Pois(P_T \lambda_{iC}); \eta_i = \lambda_{iT}/\lambda_{iC}$. For each individual AE (i^{th} AE), given the marginal total number of events for both groups ($n_i = n_{iT} + n_{iC}$) and the exposure information P_T and P_C, the count data for the treatment group (n_{iT}) and that of the control group (n_{iC}) can be created from a Multinomial (Binomial in this case) distribution, i.e., $(n_{iT}, n_{iC})|n_i \sim Multinomial(n_i; (\eta_i \frac{P_T}{\eta_i P_T + P_C}, \frac{P_C}{\eta_i P_T + P_C})), i = 1, 2, ..., I$.

Simulation steps:

- The total number of AEs ($I = 26$), the exposure information for each group ($P_T = 410.04, P_C = 203.92$), and the marginal count data of both groups for each individual AE ($n_i = (106, 154, \cdots, 14, 0)$) were set from Table 8.7.

- For type-I error evaluation, the η_i values are set to 1 for all AEs. For power evaluation, η_i is set as 1.5, 2, 5, or 8 for a specific AE to reflect the different magnitudes of the safety signal.

- To evaluate the effect of event rates (λ_{iC} and λ_{iT} in the model), especially rare event rates, on the model performance, the marginal count of the specific i^{th} AE (n_i) is modified from 20 to 200 (in this case, the reference event rate λ_{iC} is changed from 0.03 per person-year to 0.3 per person-year) while the marginal count of other AEs remain unchanged. Note that the event rate of 0.03 is obtained as $\lambda_{iC} = \lambda_{iT} = n_i/(P_T + P_C) = 20/(410.04 + 203.92) = 0.03$. It is also important to note that the event rate (adjusted by exposure time in this case) can be over 1.

- Count data for each group and each AE are generated using the above parameter settings. In each scenario, 1,000 simulations are conducted to calculate the type-I error and power.

Simulation Results

Table 8.9 presents the type-I error assessment results. The modified LRT test was found to control type-I error under the desired level (0.05) with a slight fluctuation due to the number of simulations. Given that there were 26 AEs without any multiple testing adjustment, the Z-test was unable to control the type-I error. Finally, the Z-test with BH adjustment could also control type-I error, but in a very conservative manner (< 0.05).

Table 8.10 shows the power of the three methods under different scenarios. The results suggest that either reducing the relative risk (in this case η_i) between two groups or reducing the overall event rate of both groups can potentially harm the power of the modified LRT and Z-test with BH adjustment. However, in most cases, the modified LRT appeared to be more sensitive (with higher power) than the Z-test with BH at detecting safety signals. Specifically, the modified LRT method had a rise in power from 0.097 to 0.938 when increasing the reference event rate from 0.03 per person-year to 0.3 per person-year (the total number of events ranged from 20 to 200) while maintaining the relative risk at a reasonably small level ($\eta_i = 2$). Generally, the conventional Z-test was sensitive in detecting safety signals but with inflated type-I error. The asymptotic Z-test with BH adjustment was highly conservative and lost significant power to detect signals from rare events. The simulation results indicate that the modified LRT method can control type-I error and maintain satisfactory power even in the presence of rare events.

8.3.7 Remarks

In analyzing the AE data without time at risk from Ref. [123], stroke is detected as a safety signal for HeartWare in comparison to HeartMate II, from both the modified LRT method and Z-test with BH procedure. This finding is consistent with published literature and a previous FDA safety communication ([49, 99, 123]). The p-values from the analysis with time at risk (p=0.002 and p=0.005 for LRT and Z-test with BH, respectively) are smaller than those from analysis without the time at risk (p=0.025 and p=0.027 for LRT and Z-test with BH, respectively). This indicates stronger signals when incorporating time at risk information. Given the data source, the study has only the total person-years of exposure for each device. However, more detailed exposure-time information categorized by AEs, if available, could also be analyzed using the proposed statistical methods.

Specific literature that supports stroke as a safety signal includes a recent systematic review, which found that ischemic stroke occurred in a median of 7.5% (range: 4-17.1%) of HeartWare subjects versus 6.0% (range: 0-16%) of HeartMate II subjects (Cho, Moazami, and Frontera 2017). Moreover, in a study of 734 HeartWare and HeartMate II subjects, those treated with HeartWare were found to have a higher cumulative risk of stroke (hazard ratio=1.8; 95% confidence interval: 1.25, 2.5; p=0.003) (Stulak et al. 2015). Furthermore, a retrospective cohort study of 13 HeartWare subjects and 33 HeartMate II subjects found that the probability of stroke at one year to be 44% in HeartWare vs.10% in HeartMate II (Lalonde et al. 2013).

Using Fisher's exact test to compare percentages of subjects with each AE, Rogers et al. found that the use of HeartWare is associated with more strokes ($p < 0.001$), right heart failure (0.02), and sepsis (p=0.048) as compared to those associated with the use of HeartMate II [123]. In this study, stroke is found to be a safety signal for HeartWare when compared to HeartMate II while, the other two AEs (i.e., right heart failure and sepsis) are not. This difference can be explained by the fact that both modified LRT and Z-test with BH procedure explore potential safety signals with FDR controlled, consequently resulting in fewer significant signals. The Z-test with BH procedure is used to examine AEs independently for differences in risk with p-values adjusted for multiple comparisons, while the modified LRT is built upon the global hypothesis testing that examined each AE relative to all AEs using maximization to reduce the number of false signals. Note that the LRT method can be modified to analyze the data including more than two arms in the clinical trial (such as one drug with different dose levels, different drugs, active control, and common control).

Post-market surveillance data often lacks time at risk information. While including length of exposure for individual subjects in safety surveillance provides greater insight, there are complexities in assessing the duration of device use prior to the occurrence of AEs. Following subjects implanted with devices over time poses several challenges including handling multiple payers (e.g., insurance companies), capturing the appropriate periods of time, receiving informed consent from subjects to assess their device performance, and cost. Thus, data without exact time at risk information can also provide a valuable first look and play a key role in identifying potential safety concerns for further investigation. As demonstrated through an initial application to LVADs, the proposed statistical methods can incorporate the time at risk in safety signal detection and are also capable of identifying safety signals using the number of subjects in the absence of the exposure-time information.

It is important to note that exposure information can be defined in different ways; therefore, the underlying risk for a device, or the parameter λ_i, has different clinical meanings. For example, if the exposure information is not available, P_T and P_C can be the total number of subjects in the treatment group and control group. Assuming that every patient had the same unit of time of exposure, the calculated λ is the number of subjects who experienced each AE event (as shown in Table 8.7, without time at risk). If P_T and P_C are calculated based on the time to first event, the calculated λ is exposure-adjusted incidence rate, (EAIR). For further details on different definitions of exposure, see Ref. [81].

8.3.8 Appendix: LRT and tree-based scan statistic method for comparing treatment vs. control

8.3.8.1 Summary of tree-based scan method

The purpose of the tree-based scan statistic (TBSS) method [138] is to compare the safety issues of the cases and controls (two groups). This statistic assumes that the follow-up window is the same for the exposed and comparator subjects in a matched pair and tests the null hypothesis of no difference in incidence rate for AEs in any node against a one-sided alternative that there is at least one node where the rate of AEs is higher in the exposed group than in the comparator.

The test statistic is maximum log likelihood ratio across observed nodes

$$T = max_G LLR(G),$$

and the log likelihood ratio for each node LLR(G), is based on the number of cases in the exposed or comparator group as well as the probability of being in the exposed group. Therefore,

$$LLR(G) = ln\left(\frac{(\frac{c_G}{c_G+n_G})^{c_G}(\frac{n_G}{c_G+n_G})^{n_G}}{(\rho)^{c_G}(1-\rho)^{n_G}}\right)I(\frac{c_G}{c_G+n_G} > \rho), \tag{8.2}$$

Where T = unconditional Bernoulli tree scan statistic, c_G = number of cases in the exposure group for a given node G, n_G = number of cases in the comparator group for a given node G, ρ = known probability of being in the exposure group (for 1:1 matching, ρ is 0.5).

The closed form solution for the distribution of the test statistic T under the null is unknown. For hypothesis testing using statistic T, the p-value can be derived non-parametrically using Monte Carlo simulation. Under the null, there is no association between outcomes and exposure. If the null hypothesis is true, in a 1:1 matched setting, each event within a node is equally likely to occur in either of the two treatment groups being compared (probability 0.5). In the Monte Carlo simulations, all nodes contain the same total number of events as observed in the original data. However, the exposure status is generated from a Binomial draw (probability 0.5).

The alerts (i.e., signals) can be found from 9,999 Monte Carlo simulations as follows. First, T statistics can be calculated for each of the 9,999 simulation and an additional one from the observed dataset. Then, all T statistics are ranked from largest to smallest. Finally, the p-value is the rank of the T statistic in the observed data set divided by 10,000 (9,999 simulated datasets + 1 observed dataset). With a threshold of 1%, only nodes with p-values less than 1% are alerts. Note that the threshold is the probability of an error (falsely rejecting the null).

8.3.8.2 Relationship between LRT method and tree-based scan statistic method

In addition to the unconditional TBSS method discussed in Ref. [138], the conditional TBSS method (see Section 4.5), is conditional on total number of AEs observed (and total exposure or total reports).

Therefore, under the assumption of AE counts as independent Poisson, conditional on the total $n_{.j}$ and $P_{i.}$ or $n_{i.}$, the distribution of cell counts n_{ij} is Multinomial. This is same as the TBSS, which shares the same assumptions for the AE counts used in LRT methods described in previous chapters.

The unconditional Bernoulli tree-based scan statistic (TBSS) discussed in this section assumes independent Binomial or Poisson models for AEs in two arms (case and control), such that the probability of assignment to the two arms is ρ (known from the study design, for example, 0.5).

Comparing the modified LRT described in Section 8.3.4 and the unconditional TBSS method with a pre-specified ρ, we notice that if only one layer of the adverse events is considered (such as PT terms), the c_G in 8.2 is the same as n_{iT} in 8.1 for the treatment group (Section 8.3.4) and n_G in 8.2 is the same as the n_{iC} in 8.1 for the control group (Section 8.3.4).

Both the modified LRT method discussed in Section 8.3.4, and the Bernoulli TBSS method in this section use Monte Carlo simulation for statistical inference. Both methods use the total number of events for the two groups as observed in the original data by node (or PT term).

In addition to one layer in LRT method, one can extend the LRT with one layer to LRT for multiple layers (in hierarchical structure) with index, g, including AEs or groups of AEs (discussed in Section 4.3). The test statistic will be similar for the unconditional TBSS and the modified LRT method for comparing two groups for data including more than one layer if the G in TBSS method and the g in LRT method are the same or similar for comparing the AE issues in two treatment groups with the $\rho = \frac{P_T}{P_T+P_C}$.

8.4 Spatial-Cluster Signal Detection in Medical Devices using LRT

8.4.1 Background

One of the growing interests of researchers, manufactures, and regulators in safety surveillance for medical products is to find geographic patterns of the AEs for these products. For example, an observation of a significantly higher use of a vaccine or a drug in a certain region might suggest the possibility of a foodborne disease outbreak, and further investigation may be needed to find the potential contaminated source in that area. Similarly, exploring geographic patterns for device safety in a timely manner can be helpful for alerting regulators with an early detection of safety signals, if any, associated with specific region(s). A detailed look into the problematic areas and corresponding actions can be taken immediately.

Currently, the available post-market device safety databases (e.g., Manufacturer and User Facility Device Experience (MAUDE)) [52] do not have information on the actual patient population exposed to the devices, or the device exposure-time for each patient. In a report issued by FDA in 2013 [48], four key actions are outlined to strengthen national medical device surveillance system: establish a unique device identification (UDI) system, promote the development of national medical device registries, modernize adverse event reporting and analysis, and develop and apply new methods for evidence generation, synthesis, and appraisal. Using large medical device safety data obtained from post-market surveillance, investigators can track the health outcomes of a wider patient population covering a broader geographical area for a longer period than in the premarket studies. With the development of medical device surveillance system including many registries, it is hoped that the patient-level exposure information and the geographic information will be captured in future device post-market safety databases, which will in turn make it possible, and necessary, to investigate the geographical patterns of AE risks associated with selected devices.

Several analytical approaches have been developed and used in disease surveillance for the evaluation of geographic pattern of disease incidence, including spatial scan methods [78, 94] for disease cluster detection, using data collected from registries such as Surveillance Epidemiology and End Results (SEER) Program [132]. Here, the problem of interest is a spatial-cluster signal detection for AE associated with medical devices. That is to detect clusters of spatial units (e.g., blocks, regions, counties, states, etc.) which have significantly higher AE rates compared with the rates of other geographic units in the study space, using a large post-market device safety database with exposure and geographical information. For example, we may be interested to use a database of patients with heart-disease using LVAD, to explore whether there is a spatial-cluster signal related to "stroke" (that is, if regions with higher stroke rates are geographically close to each other).

To evaluate the spatial patterns, we describe a statistical method based on likelihood ratio test (LRT), known as spatial-LRT, to detect spatial-cluster signals of medical-device-related AEs, by incorporating exposure information and geographical information. We also discuss several issues about possible usage of future post-market database in medical-device-related spatial-cluster signal detection, including variables to be collected, data format standardization, analytical method used, and the output of spatial-cluster signal for AE surveillance.

8.4.2 Spatial-LRT with exposure information

For a particular device and a fixed AE of interest, suppose that a study includes data from a total of S geographical regions. Additionally, for each region $s(s = 1, \ldots, S)$, suppose we have a pair of data (P_s, n_s), where P_s denotes the device exposure information, and n_s denotes the count of AE occurrences in region s. In this case, the study space G is defined as the entire geographical area consisting of all S geographical regions. We use a moving window to scan the study space G, such that a collection of candidate zones $Z \in G$ (Z is used to denote a subset of G) is defined, from which the spatial-cluster signal(s) (including one or several zones) can be found.

Let P_Z denote the total exposure time of device in zone Z (the sum of exposure time for all patients using the device in zone Z), P_G the total exposure time in the entire study space G, n_Z the total AE count in Z, and n_G the total AE count in G. We assume that

$$n_Z \sim Poisson(p_Z P_Z), n_G - n_Z \sim Poisson(q_Z(P_G - P_Z)),$$

and that n_Z and $n_G - n_Z$ are independent.

For a given zone Z, the likelihood ratio is

$$LR_Z = \frac{L_Z(\hat{p}_Z, \hat{q}_Z)}{L_Z(\hat{p}_0)} = \frac{\hat{p}_Z^{n_Z} \hat{q}_Z^{n_G - n_Z}}{\hat{p}_0^{n_G}}.$$

Substituting $\hat{p}_Z, \hat{q}_Z$ and $\hat{p}_0$ by the corresponding MLE, we obtain the log-likelihood ratio

$$LLR_Z = ln(LR_Z) = (n_Z)ln\frac{n_Z}{P_Z} + (n_G - n_Z)ln\frac{n_G - n_Z}{P_G - P_Z} - (n_G)ln\frac{n_G}{P_G}.$$

The test statistic for testing $H_0 : p_Z = q_Z = p_0$ for all zones, against the alternative hypothesis $H_a : p_Z > q_Z$ for at least one zone $Z \in G$, is $MLLR = max_{Z \in G} LLR_Z I(\hat{p}_Z > \hat{q}_Z)$.

There is no closed analytical form for the distribution of the test statistic. The Monte Carlo simulation is applied to construct the null distribution of the test statistic, as described in Ref. [43]. Note that, given the exposure information for each region, $P_s (s = 1, \ldots, S)$ and the total AE count n_G, the distribution of $(n_1, n_2, \ldots, n_S)$, under H_0, is a Multinomial distribution as below

$$(n_1, n_2, \ldots, n_S | n_G) \sim Multinomial(n_G, [\frac{P_1}{P_G}, \frac{P_2}{P_G}, \cdots, \frac{P_S}{P_G}]).$$

This distribution can be used to simulate MC datasets.

For each zone $Z \in G$, the observed LLR_Z is located into the empirical distribution of MLLR (obtained from the null data generated by MC procedure) and the p-value associated with that zone is determined using the formula $p - value = 100 \times (1 - (\text{rank of the observed } LLR_Z)/1000)\%$. If the null hypothesis is rejected, then we move from observed largest LLR_Z to the second largest LLR_Z, the third largest LLR_Z, and so on. The first-ranked zone is identified as the most likely cluster signal (denoted as Z_1). Among the remaining zones not geographically overlapping with zone Z_1, the first-ranked one is reported as the second most likely cluster signal, Z_2, if its p-value is smaller than α (a pre-specified threshold). We repeat this step to find the third cluster signal, the fourth cluster signal, and so on.

8.4.3 Medical device safety database considerations

To make geographical pattern exploration possible, in a database or a registry for a particular medical device of interest, the patient-level data need to include three variables; namely, geographical information s, device-exposure information P, and the AE count for health outcome of interest n. Inclusion of these variables into the medical device databases or registries may help answer future unforeseen research questions.

Data format standardization is also an important requirement for compliance with data collection, and for making the data pre-process work easier for investigators. For the device code, a unique device identification (UDI) system for medical devices was proposed by FDA in 2013 [48]. Without UDI, it is possible that one may find multiple coding ways for one device in a database obtained from registries or other sources. We provide some thoughts regarding standardizing data formats for the geographical and exposure variables.

- Geographical information s: for each patient who uses this device, geographical information can be collected from the patient (e.g., Zip code of patient's residence), from the manufacturer (e.g., an identification number of the device manufacturing site), and from the health care provider (an identification number of the provider indicating the location where the device implantation surgery is performed).

- Exposure information P: in order to obtain the exposure information, the data may include time point of device implantation, the time points of the AE occurrences, and the time points of follow-up-lost/death.

With available exposure and geographical variables, and a clearly-defined health outcome (AE) of interest available in the registries, the spatial-LRT can be conveniently implemented to explore spatial-cluster pattern for device-related AEs.

8.4.4 Illustrations

We illustrate the method using two hypothetical cases where data are generated over 48 states in US mainland regarding LVAD, a medical device class used for heart diseases [53, 135]. Case 1 illustrates an example with a single target cluster of irregular shape, and Case 2 illustrates an example with two target clusters.

Case 1 includes a single cluster signal (true signal) with a diagonal (irregular) shape from West US to Northeast US, consisting of 10 connected states (AZ, NM, OK, MO, KY, IN, WV, MD, PA, and NY). Case 2 includes 2 cluster signals (true signals) with 4 connected states in West US (AZ, NM, CO, UT) and 6 connected states in Northeast US (ME, NH, VT, MA, RI, and CT).

The AE rate for stroke is set to be 0.1 (representing low rate) for the area outside the cluster(s); and 0.3 (representing high rate) for the area inside the cluster(s). The information for the AE rates in different LVAD devices can be found in summaries of safety and effectiveness data(https://www.accessdata.fda.gov/scripts/cdrh/cfdocs/cfpma/pma.cfm). The estimated total number of patients in U.S. using LVADs in 2014 (3795 from Ref. [26]) are assigned to each state by a Multinomial distribution with the fixed total $P_G = 3795$.

For each of 48 states in US mainland, the hypothetical data are comprised of the total number of LVAD use in the state and the related number of stroke occurrences associated with LVAD use. The LRT results for the two cases are summarized below.

For Case 1, the number of LVAD use in the states ranges from 52 to 113. The total number of strokes (n_G) is 502 out of 3670 LVAD uses, and the observed nation-wide incidence rate from the data is 13.68% (502/3670). We searched for connected regions containing up to 14 candidate states in US mainland.

To ease the interpretation of the detected signal(s), we suggest embedding a table summarizing AE incidence rate, LLR and p-value for each cluster signal, and a map visualizing the cluster distribution, into the output from the statistical tool. See Table 8.11 and Figure 8.3 for the analysis results of Case 1. In Figure 8.3, the most likely cluster signal detected with the LRT method is marked in green (consisting of the states of Arizona, New Mexico, Oklahoma, Missouri, Kentucky, Indiana, Michigan, West Virginia, Maryland, Pennsylvania, and New York). The detected cluster is a narrow zone stretching from west to northeast, which is difficult to find with circular or square moving windows. The AE incidence is 0.255 (95% CI: 0.254–0.256) inside, and 0.100 (95% CI: 0.0999–0.1001) outside the detected spatial-cluster. Compared with the true cluster pattern, the detected signal is mostly consistent with the true pattern, except that Michigan is erroneously included into the cluster.

For Case 2, the number of LVAD use in the states ranges from 37–117. The total number of strokes (n_G) is 499 out of 3643 LVAD uses, which gives an observed nation-wide incidence rate 13.70% (499/3643). Figure 8.4 shows that two cluster signals are detected (cluster A marked in green and cluster B marked in blue area). The most likely cluster signal A consists of 6 states in the Northeast including Maine, Connecticut, Rhode Island, Massachusetts, New Hampshire, and Vermont. The secondary cluster signal B comprises 3 states in the West including Arizona, Colorado, and Utah. The AE incidence is 0.325 (95% CI: 0.323–0.327) for cluster A, 0.307 (95% CI: 0.303–0.311) for cluster B, and 0.102 (95% CI: 0.1019–0.1021) for the rest of the areas (Table 8.12). In comparison with the true cluster pattern, the detected signal is mostly consistent with the true pattern, except that New Mexico state is not detected as a part of cluster A.

8.4.5 Remarks

In post-market safety surveillance, it is important to identify safety issues using medical device databases/registries covering large geographical regions. Note that in the proposed statistical method, the geographical region can be defined as a spatial unit at any level, such as clinical sites, blocks, regions, counties, states, countries, etc. A spatial-cluster signal is a zone consisting of multiple connective regions with a significantly higher AE rate compared with rates of other regions regarding a specific device. Although the outcome of interest is an AE count in our problem setting, the method can be applied to any count outcomes.

The computational burden of the method may be affected by the size of the cluster signal and the shape of the moving window. For example, the computational time may increase substantially if a flexible-shaped window is used for a large spatial-cluster pattern. The appropriate strategies to reduce the number of candidate clusters are usually applied in such cases [40, 98]. Filtering and partitioning are commonly used approaches in graph mining to drop false candidates in early screening stage [103, 148], and can be easily engineered into our method. For example, one can filter regions with an AE risk lower than a pre-specified threshold to reduce the searching space. One can also partition the entire study space into several smaller spaces, and search for the spatial-cluster signal within each smaller space. Attempts may also be made to extend the spatial LRT method to allow the inclusion of other covariates if the related information is available in a device database. We can also monitor the geographical pattern changes over time, when a dynamic device safety database becomes available (i.e., the data updates over time).

8.5 Weighted LRT Method to Device Data From Multiple Sites

8.5.1 Background

In this section, the basic LRT method (details in Chapter 3) and weighted LRT method (details in Chapter 7) are applied to the two device data (including multiple studies) discussed in the executive summary for the panel meeting (https://www.fda.gov/media/127698/download) and in Katsanos et al. [87]. One dataset (Data A) includes four studies in FDA's primary analysis with a 5-year follow-up (discussed in the executive summary), and another dataset (Data B) includes 12 studies with 2-year follow-up (in Ref. [87]).

FDA provides the results of a patient-level meta-analysis in the Executive Summary for the General Issues Panel Meeting on the late mortality safety signal associated with paclitaxel-coated products (i.e., paclitaxel-coated balloons and paclitaxeleluting stents) used to treat peripheral arterial disease in the femoropopliteal arteries (https://www.fda.gov/media/127698/download).

This panel meeting was held to review the available information and provide feedback on issues including the presence and magnitude of a late mortality safety signal, whether all paclitaxel-coated vascular products (regardless of device platform or dose) are associated with the signal, the impact of the signal on ongoing femoropopliteal disease clinical trials, and others.

FDA's primary analysis of patient-level data was limited to the four pivotal randomized control trials (RCTs) of paclitaxel (PTX)-coated devices versus non-paclitaxel (PTX)-coated devices that supported premarket approval (PMA) applications. The four pivotal RCTs with US/outside the United States (OUS) sites and 5 year follow-up are (1) S1: ZILVER PTX RCT; (2) S2: LEVANT 2; (3) S3: IN.PACT SFA I & II; and (4) S4: ILLUMENATE.

Studies S1, S2, and S3 all had five year follow-up completed, and Study S4 had three year follow-up completed at the time of the panel meeting.

The safety analysis is based on As-Treated (AT) Population, in which the treatment group assignment is based on the actual treatment a subject received during the index procedure (after the randomization, if applicable). The data information can be found in the summary file, Table 7, and Figures 11–14 (https://www.fda.gov/media/127698/download).

Katsanos et al. [87] performed a systematic review and meta-analysis of RCTs investigating paclitaxel-coated devices in the femoral and/or popliteal arteries. One analysis is based on a 2-yr dataset of 12 studies shown in Figure 2 (in Ref. [87]) including a random-effects forest plot and event information. In all, 12 studies reported the incidence of all-cause patient death up to 2 years in a total of 2316 patients. There was strong evidence that application of paclitaxel-coated devices in the femoropopliteal artery was related to significantly increased risk of death [87].

8.5.2 Data structure for data with multiple studies

Suppose there are I treatment arms, for each treatment arm, i, there are S_i studies, and one AE j^* evaluated. The objective is to find whether there is any treatment arm with a higher AE rate than other treatment arms for data combined from all studies. As a special case, the dataset has only 2 arms, i.e., treatment and control ($I = 2$). The general data structure of each study s is shown in Table 8.13 for a specific years follow-up (for example, 2 years follow-up).

$I = 2$ for both Data A and Data B. For Data A, S=4 whereas for Data B, S=12. The AE of interest is all cause mortality. The n_{ijs} is the mortality count for ith treatment and sth study; and P_{is} is considered as the number of evaluable patients for ith treatment and sth study. These data including the n_{ijs} and P_{is} can be generated for each dataset with 1-year, 2-year, 3-year, 4-year, and 5-year follow-up.

8.5.3 Weighted LRT method

The weighted LRT method (wLRT) for analyzing data with multiple studies for drugs is discussed in Chapter 7.

The hypothesis and the method for this device application are summarized below.

Hypothesis-testing for weighted LRT method $H_0 : p_i = q_i = p_0$ for all i. vs. $H_a : p_i > q_i$ for at least one $i, i = 1, \cdots, I$, p_i is the event rate of row i averaged across studies for i, ie, S_i; q_i is the event rate of all the other rows except i, when averaged across the corresponding studies.

Statistic for Weighted LRT method (wLR)

Step 1

For each study s and each row i, calculate $log(LR_{ijs})$ using the basic LRT method

$$log(LR_{ijs}) = log((\frac{n_{ijs}}{P_{is}})^{n_{ijs}}(\frac{n_{.js} - n_{ijs}}{P_{.s} - P_{is}})^{n_{.js}-n_{ijs}}/(\frac{n_{.js}}{P_{.s}})^{n_{.js}}). \tag{8.3}$$

Step 2

For each row i (treatment arm i), calculate weighted average of $log(LR_{ijs})$ S_i. S_i is the number of studies for treatment/row i.

$$wLR_{ij} = \frac{\sum_{s=1}^{S_i} P_{is} log(LR_{ijs})}{\sum_{s=1}^{S_i} P_{is}}, \tag{8.4}$$

where wLR_{ij} is the observed test statistic for each row i in the presence of multiple studies.

Step 3

Calculate the maximum of wLR_{ij} among all treatment arms/rows.

$$MwLR = max_i(wLR_{ij}). \tag{8.5}$$

Step 4 (calculate p-value through simulation)

Use Monte Carlo method to build the empirical distribution of $MwLR$ under null hypothesis. For each study s, one can generate $(n_{1js}, \cdots, n_{Ijs}) \sim multi(n_{.js}, (\frac{P_{1s}}{\sum_{i=1}^{I} P_{is}}, \cdots, \frac{P_{Is}}{\sum_{i=1}^{I} P_{is}}))$, independently. The $MwLR$ is calculated for each generated dataset using the above mentioned step 1–3.

8.5.4 Results

Results from applications of the weight LRT method are shown in Table 8.14 for Data A analysis and Table 8.15 for Data B analysis.

Since Data A has data with up to 5 year follow-up, the analysis is conducted for the data with 1-year, 2-year, 3-year, 4-year, and 5-year follow-up separately.

As shown in Table 8.14, the results of analyses of year 1, year 2, and year 3 data, which consist of four pivotal RCTs, show a trend of an increasing significance with overall p-values (from the weighted LRT method for multiple studies) changing from 0.3383 to 0.02 for the paclitaxel-coated device signal, which is consistent with the results from relative risk analysis provided in Table 7 and Figures 11–13 in the executive summary (https://www.fda.gov/media/127698/download). The p-value stays low (0.009) for the analysis of the year 5 data with less studies. To be conservative, one may compare the p-values from the analysis over time (Data A) with $\alpha(k) = \alpha/2^k$ (details in Section 6.3).

As shown in Table 8.15, the overall p-value from the weighted LRT method is 0.016 for Data B with 12 studies, which is consistent with the overall results shown in the random effect forest analysis ([87]) and can support the signal of paclitaxel-coated device for mortality as AE of interest. For individual study analysis using LRT method, we notice that the LRT method identified one individual study with p-values$<$ 0.5 (IN.PACT SFA) and the random forest analysis indicates that only study IN.PACT SFA has the 95% confidence interval of the relative risk $>$ 1.

8.5.5 Remarks

Applications of LRT and weighted LRT methods on the device data including multiple studies are discussed in this section.

Individual studies may not have statistical significance for safety evaluation (shown in the above two examples). However, if the results from individual studies are consistent, the analysis by combining the information from all the studies may show signals of safety issues with significance.

The results from the traditional meta-analysis using random forest plot for relative risk and random effect model or fixed effect model are consistent with the results from LRT method (basic LRT for individual study and weighted LRT for all studies together). In the illustration, there are two arms in the studies (treatment vs. control). If there are more than two arms in the study,

LRT method can also be used with overall type-I error controlled. However, the traditional meta-analysis is not designed for studies with more than two arms.

8.6 Tables and Figures

FIGURE 8.1
Stacked Venn diagram of the safety signals detected by different methods.

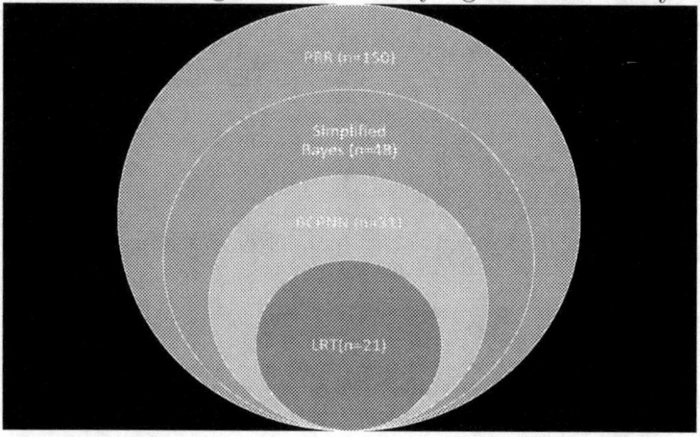

FIGURE 8.2
LRT exploration over years for top five AEs in HeartMate II.

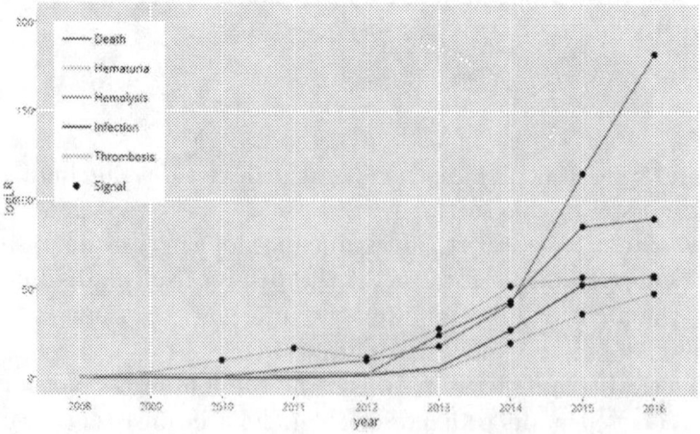

FIGURE 8.3
Cluster of high stroke rate for LVAD in US mainland detected, Case 1.

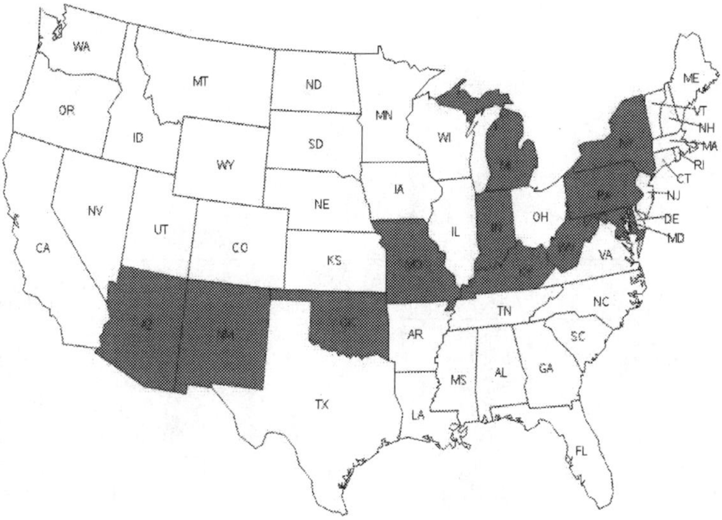

FIGURE 8.4
Cluster signals of high stroke rate for LVAD in US mainland detected, Case 2.

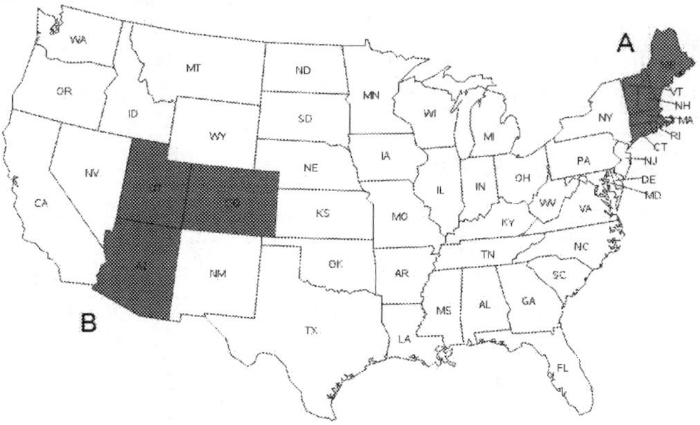

TABLE 8.1
AE signals detected by the LRT method for HeartMate II.

Type of AE	Reported AE counts HeartMate II only	All LVADs	RR	logLR	p-value
Hemolysis	4428	5914	1.92	711.72	0
Complaint, Ill-Defined	920	1037	2.19	218.24	0
Death	4704	8628	1.37	191.04	0
Thrombus	4538	8732	1.3	129.51	0
Hemorrhage, cerebral	1061	1635	1.6	98.4	0
Enzyme Elevation, Cardiac	327	349	2.3	86.8	0
Infarction, cerebral	632	948	1.64	64.67	0
Dyspnea	559	871	1.57	49.13	0
Wound Infection, Post-Operative	623	1039	1.47	40.32	0
Hematuria	640	1097	1.43	36	0
Thrombosis	626	1100	1.39	30.67	0
Cardiac Arrest	265	474	1.37	11.61	0.0002
Infection	2031	4467	1.11	11.03	0.0005
Syncope	337	642	1.28	9.58	0.0019
Heart Failure	679	1407	1.18	8.71	0.0049
Chest Pain	188	342	1.34	7.39	0.0173
Aortic insufficiency	110	184	1.46	6.95	0.0258
Hemorrhage, Subarachnoid	151	271	1.36	6.46	0.0427

RR is relative reporting rate. There are more than 300 AE terms (LLT/PT terms) in the data. Only AE terms with p-value<0.05 *(excluding "no information", "no code", "not applicable", "test") are shown in the table with logLR values from largest to smallest ones.*

TABLE 8.2
AE signals detected by PRR, sB, and BCPNN for HeartMate II.

Type of AE	Reported AE counts HeartMate II only	All LVADs	Low_{RR}	Low_{IC95}	Low_{sB05}
Complaint, Ill-Defined	920	1037	2.14	0.98	2.02
Enzyme Elevation, Cardiac	327	349	2.23	0.97	2.03
Hemolysis	4428	5914	1.88	0.81	1.77
Infarction, cerebral	632	948	1.56	0.55	1.50
Hemorrhage, cerebral	1061	1635	1.54	0.55	1.49
Dyspnea	559	871	1.50	0.49	1.44
Wound Infection, Post-Operative	623	1039	1.40	0.40	1.35
Hematuria	640	1097	1.36	0.37	1.31
Death	4704	8628	1.34	0.36	1.29
Thrombosis	626	1100	1.32	0.33	1.28
Thrombus	4538	8732	1.27	0.29	1.23
Cardiac Arrest	265	474	1.26	0.23	1.20
Aortic insufficiency	110	184	1.30	0.19	1.18
Coma	28	35	1.65	0.17	1.22
Edema	83	136	1.30	0.16	1.17
Syncope	337	642	1.19	0.16	1.14
Chest Pain	188	342	1.22	0.16	1.15
Therapeutic Response, Decreased	27	34	1.63	0.15	1.19
Hemorrhage, Subarachnoid	151	271	1.22	0.15	1.14
Pain	199	377	1.17	0.11	1.11
Heart Failure	679	1407	1.12	0.10	1.09
Fall	132	244	1.18	0.09	1.09
Fatigue	230	450	1.14	0.09	1.09
Infection	2031	4467	1.08	0.07	1.06
Vascular System (Circulation)	33	48	1.39	0.06	1.10
Congestive Heart Failure	65	113	1.20	0.03	1.06
Hemorrhage, Subdural	78	140	1.17	0.03	1.06
Shock, Cardiogenic	121	232	1.13	0.02	1.05

$Lower_{RR}$ is the lower bound of the 95% Confidence Interval for RR. An AE with a $Lower_{RR}$ greater than 1 is considered as a possible signal. Low_{IC95} stands for the lower bound of the 95% credible interval for the BCPNN method. If the Low_{IC95} is greater than 0, the corresponding AE is an AE signal. $Low_{sB0.5}$ represents the lower bound of the 95% credible interval of the simplified Bayes method with c = 0.5. If the $Low_{sB0.5}$ is greater than 1, the corresponding AE is an AE signal. Only AE terms with $Low_{IC95} > 0$ are shown in the table. The AE signals are ordered by their logLR values.

TABLE 8.3
AE signals including SOCs detected by LRT method for HeartMate II.

	Reported AE counts				
Type of AE	HeartMate II only	All LVADs	RR	logLR	p-value
Hemolysis (in BLS)	4428	5914	1.92	711.72	0
Blood and lymphatic system disorders (BLS SOC)	4769	6728	1.82	649.38	0
Complaint, Ill-defined	920	1037	2.19	218.24	0
Death	4704	8628	1.37	191.04	0
Thrombus	4538	8732	1.30	129.51	0
Hemorrhage, cerebral	1061	1635	1.60	98.40	0
Enzyme elevation, cardiac	327	349	2.30	86.80	0
Infarction, cerebral	632	948	1.64	64.67	0
Dyspnea (in CD)	559	871	1.57	49.13	0
Wound infection, post-operative	623	1039	1.47	40.32	0
Hematuria	640	1097	1.43	36.0	0
Thrombosis	626	1100	1.39	30.67	0
Cardiac disorders (CD SOC)	3341	7500	1.09	12.14	0.0002
Cardiac arrest (in CD)	265	474	1.37	11.61	00003
Infection	2031	4467	1.11	11.03	0.0004
Syncope (in CD)	337	642	1.28	9.58	0.0022
Heart failure (in CD)	679	1407	1.18	8.71	0.0048
Chest pain (in CD)	188	342	1.34	7.39	0.017
Aortic insufficiency	110	184	1.46	6.95	0.0243
Hemorrhage, subarachnoid	151	271	1.36	6.46	0.0419

RR is relative reporting rate. Only AE terms with p-value<0.05 (excluding "no information", "no code", "not applicable") are shown in the table, and are ordered by logLR values.

TABLE 8.4
AE signals of device problem codes, detected by LRT method for HeartMate II.

Type of AE	Reported AE counts HeartMate II only	All LVADs	RR	logLR	p-value
Device stops intermittently	1424	1501	1.84	209.65	0
High Readings	1122	1136	1.91	184.81	0
Infusion or flow issue	1375	1528	1.74	170.15	0
Break	608	660	1.76	79.69	0
Decreased pump speed	505	528	1.82	74.37	0
Occlusion within device	563	678	1.58	50.32	0
Electrical shorting	283	288	1.87	44.93	0
Malposition of device	276	309	1.7	32.28	0
Use of device issue	225	254	1.68	25.52	0
Blockage within device or device component	148	156	1.8	21.05	0
Device operates differently than expected	969	1536	1.2	14.66	0
Disconnection	268	370	1.37	12.05	0.0002
Migration of device or device component	74	77	1.82	10.93	0.0007
Maintenance does not comply to manufacturers recommendations	65	65	1.89	10.79	0.0007
Kinked	94	113	1.57	8.35	0.0042
Noise, audible	77	91	1.6	7.32	0.0129
Vibration	45	46	1.85	7.01	0.0187
Power conditioning issue	100	127	1.49	6.98	0.0201
Motor drive unit	110	145	1.44	6.38	0.0371

RR is relative reporting rate. There are a total of more than 200 AE terms (device problem codes) in the data. Only AE terms with p-value$<$ 0.05 *(excluding "other", "no information", "no code", "not applicable") are shown in the table, and are ordered by logLR values.*

TABLE 8.5
Safety signal assessment comparing HeartWare and HeartMate II without and with time at risk.

	Treatment group HeartWare ($n = 296$)[a]	Control group HeartMate II ($n = 149$)[a]	P-value for analysis without time at risk		P-value for analysis with time at risk[b]	
Adverse event	# of patients with events	# of patients with events	modified LRT	Z-test with BH	modified LRT	Z-test with BH
Stroke	88	18	0.025	0.027	0.002	0.005
Right heart failure	114	40	0.994	0.575	0.663	0.343
Sepsis	70	23	0.996	0.575	0.805	0.343
Transient ischemic attack	25	7	0.999	0.575	0.982	0.361
Aortic valve incompetence	3	0	1.000	0.575	1.000	0.396
Arterial thromboembolism	18	10	1.000	0.988	1.000	0.848
Bleeding events	178	90	1.000	0.988	1.000	0.848
Cardiac arrhythmia	112	61	1.000	0.988	1.000	0.942
Cardiac tamponade	0	1	1.000	0.988	1.000	0.960
Death	116	48	1.000	0.861	0.999	0.426
Device lead damage	2	2	1.000	0.988	1.000	0.953
Device malfunction or failure	93	38	1.000	0.861	0.999	0.426
Drive-line exit-site infection	58	23	1.000	0.861	1.000	0.446
Hemolysis	24	13	1.000	0.988	1.000	0.848
Hepatic dysfunction	14	12	1.000	0.988	1.000	0.960
Hypertension	47	25	1.000	0.988	1.000	0.848
Localized non-device infection	148	65	1.000	0.949	1.000	0.458
Multi-organ failure	6	6	1.000	0.988	1.000	0.960
Myocardial infarction	4	0	1.000	0.575	1.000	0.361
Psychiatric	48	16	1.000	0.575	0.977	0.361
Pump replacement	23	20	1.000	0.988	1.000	0.968
Rehospitalization	249	118	1.000	0.988	1.000	0.595
Renal dysfunction	44	18	1.000	0.880	1.000	0.505
Respiratory dysfunction	86	38	1.000	0.949	1.000	0.523
Thrombocytopenia	7	7	1.000	0.988	1.000	0.960
Wound dehiscence	0	0	1.000	NA^c	1.000	NA^c
Total	1,577	699				

LRT = likelihood ratio test; BH = Benjamini-Hochberg procedure; NA = not applicable. a: The number of patients with each adverse event for HeartWare and HeartMate II were previously published in Table 3 and Table S13 of [123] b: 410 patient-years were evaluated for HeartWare, and 204 patients-years were evaluated for HeartMate II. c: The p-values for the Z-test with BH were NA due to there being zero patients with wound dehiscence for both devices.

TABLE 8.6
Safety signal assessment comparing HeartWare and HeartMate II without and with time at risk including two SOCs.

	Treatment group HeartWare ($n = 296$)	Control group HeartMate II ($n = 149$)	P-value for analysis without time at risk	with time at risk
Adverse event	# of patients with events	# of patients with events	modified LRT	modified LRT
Stroke	88	18	0.033	0.003
Pump replacement	23	20	0.515	0.793
Hepatic dysfunction	14	12	0.929	0.983
Thrombocytopenia (in BLS)	7	7	0.971	0.989
blood and lymphatic system disorders (BLS SOC)	209	110	0.975	1
Multi organ failure	6	6	0.987	0.997
Right heart failure (in CD)	114	40	0.994	0.682
Cardiac arrhythmia (in CD)	112	61	0.996	1
Sepsis	70	23	0.997	0.818
Bleeding events (in BLS)	178	90	1	1
Hypertension	47	25	1	1
Drive-line exit site infection	58	23	1	1
Transient ischemic attack	25	7	1	0.98
Renal dysfunction	44	18	1	1
Respiratory dysfunction	86	38	1	1
Device malfunction or failure	93	38	1	1
Rehospitalization	249	118	1	1
Death	116	48	1	1
Aortic valve incompetence (in CD)	3	0	1	1
Cardiac tamponade (in CD)	0	1	1	1
Myocardial infarction (in CD)	4	0	1	1
Localized non device infection	148	65	1	1
Psychiatric	48	16	1	0.977
Arterial thromboembolism	18	10	1	1
Wound dehiscence	0	0	1	1
Hemolysis (in BLS)	24	13	1	1
Device lead damage	2	2	1	1
cardiac disorders (CD SOC)	233	102	1	1

TABLE 8.7
Safety signal assessment comparing HeartWare and HeartMate II without and with time at risk.

	Treatment group HeartWare ($n = 296$)[a]	Control group HeartMate II ($n = 149$)[a]	P-value for analysis without time at risk		with time at risk[b]	
Adverse event	# of patients with events	# of patients with events	modified LRT	Z-test with BH	modified LRT	Z-test with BH
Stroke	88	18	0.025	0.027	0.002	0.005
Right heart failure	114	40	0.994	0.575	0.663	0.343
Sepsis	70	23	0.996	0.575	0.805	0.343
Transient ischemic attack	25	7	0.999	0.575	0.982	0.361
Aortic valve incompetence	3	0	1.000	0.575	1.000	0.396
Arterial thromboembolism	18	10	1.000	0.988	1.000	0.848
Bleeding events	178	90	1.000	0.988	1.000	0.848
Cardiac arrhythmia	112	61	1.000	0.988	1.000	0.942
Cardiac tamponade	0	1	1.000	0.988	1.000	0.960
Death	116	48	1.000	0.861	0.999	0.426
Device lead damage	2	2	1.000	0.988	1.000	0.953
Device malfunction or failure	93	38	1.000	0.861	0.999	0.426
Drive-line exit-site infection	58	23	1.000	0.861	1.000	0.446
Hemolysis	24	13	1.000	0.988	1.000	0.848
Hepatic dysfunction	14	12	1.000	0.988	1.000	0.960
Hypertension	47	25	1.000	0.988	1.000	0.848
Localized non-device infection	148	65	1.000	0.949	1.000	0.458
Multi-organ failure	6	6	1.000	0.988	1.000	0.960
Myocardial infarction	4	0	1.000	0.575	1.000	0.361
Psychiatric	48	16	1.000	0.575	0.977	0.361
Pump replacement	23	20	1.000	0.988	1.000	0.968
Rehospitalization	249	118	1.000	0.988	1.000	0.595
Renal dysfunction	44	18	1.000	0.880	1.000	0.505
Respiratory dysfunction	86	38	1.000	0.949	1.000	0.523
Thrombocytopenia	7	7	1.000	0.988	1.000	0.960
Wound dehiscence	0	0	1.000	NA^c	1.000	NA^c
Total	1,577	699				

LRT = likelihood ratio test; BH = Benjamini-Hochberg procedure; NA = not applicable. a: The number of patients with each adverse event for HeartWare and HeartMate II were previously published in Table 3 and Table S13 of [123] b: 410 patient-years were evaluated for HeartWare, and 204 patients-years were evaluated for HeartMate II. c: The p-values for the Z-test with BH were NA due to there being zero patients with wound dehiscence for both devices.

TABLE 8.8
Safety signal Assessment Comparing HeartWare and HeartMate II without and with time at risk including two SOCs.

	Treatment group HeartWare ($n = 296$)	Control group HeartMate II ($n = 149$)	P-value for analysis without time at risk	with time at risk
Adverse event	# of patients with events	# of patients with events	modified LRT	modified LRT
Stroke	88	18	0.033	0.003
Pump replacement	23	20	0.515	0.793
Hepatic dysfunction	14	12	0.929	0.983
Thrombocytopenia (in BLS)	7	7	0.971	0.989
blood and lymphatic system disorders (BLS SOC)	209	110	0.975	1
Multi organ failure	6	6	0.987	0.997
Right heart failure (in CD)	114	40	0.994	0.682
Cardiac arrhythmia (in CD)	112	61	0.996	1
Sepsis	70	23	0.997	0.818
Bleeding events (in BLS)	178	90	1	1
Hypertension	47	25	1	1
Drive-line exit site infection	58	23	1	1
Transient ischemic attack	25	7	1	0.98
Renal dysfunction	44	18	1	1
Respiratory dysfunction	86	38	1	1
Device malfunction or failure	93	38	1	1
Rehospitalization	249	118	1	1
Death	116	48	1	1
Aortic valve incompetence (in CD)	3	0	1	1
Cardiac tamponade (in CD)	0	1	1	1
Myocardial infarction (in CD)	4	0	1	1
Localized non device infection	148	65	1	1
Psychiatric	48	16	1	0.977
Arterial thromboembolism	18	10	1	1
Wound dehiscence	0	0	1	1
Hemolysis (in BLS)	24	13	1	1
Device lead damage	2	2	1	1
cardiac disorders (CD SOC)	233	102	1	1

TABLE 8.9
Simulation results: Type-I error assessment for cases with $\eta_i = 1$ for all AEs.

Total number of subjects with with a specific event n_i	Modified LRT test	Asymptotic Z-test	Z-test with BH adjustment
20	0.055	0.633	0.023
50	0.043	0.643	0.018
60	0.052	0.66	0.03
80	0.044	0.647	0.022
100	0.047	0.63	0.022
150	0.047	0.646	0.024
200	0.045	0.651	0.025

TABLE 8.10
Simulation results: Power assessment.

Total number of subjects with with a specific event n_i	Modified LRT test	Asymptotic Z-test	Z-test with BH adjustment
$\eta_i = 1.5$			
20	0.072	0.717	0.027
50	0.11	0.798	0.075
80	0.162	0.812	0.103
100	0.189	0.846	0.119
150	0.311	0.905	0.232
200	0.443	0.94	0.376
$\eta_i = 2$			
20	0.097	0.798	0.038
50	0.207	0.896	0.184
100	0.619	0.977	0.511
150	0.819	0.988	0.76
200	0.938	0.998	0.916
$\eta_i = 5$			
20	0.335	0.967	0.194
50	0.917	0.998	0.916
100	1	1	0.999
150	1	1	1
200	1	1	1
$\eta_i = 8$			
20	0.412	0.99	0.319
50	0.95	1	0.993
100	0.994	1	1
150	1	1	1
200	1	1	1

TABLE 8.11
The summary results for the (single) detected spatial-cluster signal, case 1.

# AEs	# devices used	Incidence (95% CI)	LLR	p-value
221	866	0.255 (0.254, 0.256)	50.402	0.002

TABLE 8.12
The summary results for the detected spatial-cluster signals, Case 2.

cluster	# AEs	# subjects	Incidence (95% CI)	LLR	p-value
A	137	422	0.325 (0.323, 0.327)	46.6	0.000
B	51	166	0.307 (0.303, 0.311)	13.8	0.001

TABLE 8.13
Data structure for a specific study s with a fixed year follow-up.

Arms (I)	# of events for AE j	Exposure information
1	n_{1js}	P_{1s}
	...	
I	n_{ijs}	P_{is}
Total	$n_{.js}$	$P_{.s}$

TABLE 8.14
Basic LRT for each study and weighted LRT for multiple studies.

		Treatment group		Control group					
Year	studies	#events	total	#events	total	rr (95% CI)	obsstat	95% threshold	p-value
1-yr	S1	8	287	4	162	1.13 (0.35, 3.69)	0.02	2.31	0.9949
1-yr	S2	6	296	4	149	0.76 (0.22, 2.63)	0	1.51	1
1-yr	S3	4	209	0	107	4.62 (0.25, 84.98)	1.65	1.41	0
1-yr	S4	4	196	1	99	2.02 (0.23, 17.84)	0.23	0.73	0.5452
1-yr	wLRT-overall	22	988	9	517	1.25 (0.59, 2.65)	0.40	0.82	0.3383
2-yr	S1	18	264	8	146	1.24 (0.55, 2.79)	0.14	1.79	0.6929
2-yr	S2	19	285	8	146	1.22 (0.55, 2.71)	0.11	1.84	0.6998
2-yr	S3	16	204	1	104	8.16 (1.10, 60.66)	3.87	2.19	0.0097
2-yr	S4	13	185	7	95	0.95 (0.39, 2.31)	0	1.86	1
2-yr	wLRT-overall	66	938	24	491	1.44 (0.91, 2.27)	0.91	1.04	0.0733
3-yr	S1	31	241	12	133	1.43 (0.76, 2.68)	0.57	2.18	0.3517
3-yr	S2	28	277	9	140	1.57 (0.76, 3.24)	0.75	1.97	0.2397
3-yr	S3	21	195	2	101	5.44 (1.30, 22.73)	4.12	1.60	0.0074
3-yr	S4	17	156	10	77	0.84 (0.40, 1.74)	0	2.02	1
3-yr	wLRT-overall	97	869	33	451	1.53 (1.05, 2.23)	1.32	1.04	0.0201
5-yr	S1	48	185	16	111	1.80 (1.08, 3.01)	2.26	2.07	0.041
5-yr	S2	54	266	17	137	1.64 (0.99, 2.71)	1.70	1.86	0.0825
5-yr	S3	30	178	9	94	1.76 (0.87, 3.55)	1.22	1.85	0.1405
5-yr	wLRT-overall	132	629	42	342	1.72 (1.25, 2.37)	1.73	1.16	0.0094

The events, totals, relative risk (rr) are obtained from in the executive summary for the panel meeting (https://www.fda.gov/media/127698/download). The confidence intervals for the overall row is from fixed effect model. obsstat for the wLRT method is described in Equation 8.5. obsstat for the individual studies is $max_i(logLR_{ijs}), i = 1, 2$, *for a particular* s. *The threshold is the 95th percentile of the empirical distribution of the statistics for basic LRT or weighted LRT methods.*

TABLE 8.15
Basic LRT for each study and weighted LRT for multiple studies for Data B including 12 studies with 2-years follow-up.

studies	Pacitaxel		Control		rr (95%CI)	obsstat	95% threshold	p-value
	event	total	event	total				
ZILVER-PTX	19	297	7	177	1.62(0.69, 3.77)	0.633	2.014	0.320
FINN-PTX	1	23	0	18	2.36(0.10, 54.68)	0.000	0.000	1.000
IN.PACT SFA	16	198	1	106	8.57(1.15, 63.70)	4.111	2.020	0.009
FEMPAC	7	45	3	42	2.18(0.60, 7.88)	0.691	2.140	0.340
LEVANT I	4	49	5	52	0.85(0.24, 2.98)	0.000	1.623	1.000
LEVANT II	21	278	7	140	1.51(0.66, 3.47)	0.477	1.712	0.426
CONSEQUENT	2	70	1	65	1.86(0.17, 20.00)	0.135	0.209	0.750
ILLUMINATE EU	13	199	3	59	1.28(0.38, 4.36)	0.081	1.700	0.762
ISAR-STATH	3	48	1	107	6.69(0.71, 62.66)	1.638	1.638	0.077
ISAR-PEBIS	3	28	0	29	7.25(0.39, 134.09)	0.000	0.188	1.000
ACOART I	8	96	6	95	1.32(0.48, 3.66)	0.133	2.388	0.798
IN.PACT SFA JAPAN	4	66	1	29	1.76(0.21, 15.05)	0.141	0.923	0.528
wLRT-overall	101	1397	35	919	1.84(1.27, 2.68)	0.925	0.708	0.016

The events, totals, relative risk (rr) are obtained from Ref. [87]. The confidence intervals for the overall row is from fixed effect model. obsstat for the wLRT method is described in Equation 8.5. obsstat for the individual studies is $max_i(logLR_{ijs}), i = 1, 2,$ *for a particular s. The threshold is the 95th percentile of the empirical distribution of the statistics for basic LRT or weighted LRT methods.*

9

LRT Method for Multiple-Site Device Data with Continuous Outcomes

9.1 Background

This chapter describes the LRT method proposed by Hu et. al. [76] for data with continuous outcomes and multiple sites. The medical device industry is one of the most rapidly growing areas in medical innovation development [89] in recent decades. FDA was authorized to build performance standards and apply inspection/recall mechanisms to monitor medical device products since 1971 [111]. With thousands of new medical devices cleared every year [29, 89], there is a fast-growing interest in understanding the performance of devices on the market. Studies have evaluated performance of a single type of medical device (e.g., [62, 118]). However, there is a lack of methodology to explore the performances of multiple medical devices simultaneously using data from multiple sources. For example, in the presence of multiple devices approved in the market for similar indications, one may want to compare devices and identify device signals by using data from different registries (sites) for different device classes.

Given a study for multiple devices conducted in multiple sites (or regions), the problem of interest is to detect if any device performs significantly differently from other devices regarding the outcome of interest. Note that the device output could be count data (e.g., number of adverse events for safety issues, number of inappropriate shocks of an implantable cardioverter defibrillator, etc.) or continuous data (e.g., blood pressure, weight loss for obesity treatment, hemoglobin A1c level for diabetes, Brain Natriuretic Peptide (BNP) level associated with heart failure, Prostate Specific Antigen (PSA) levels for prostate cancers, etc.).

One approach is to directly pool data from all sites for analysis and compare multiple devices. However, analysis based on such simple data pooling strategy may be biased, considering the potential heterogeneity of data among sites. Recently, some novel analytical approaches have been developed for count data evaluation with multiple sites [142] and/or multiple studies [82]. However, when the outcome of interest is a continuous variable, these methods, which were developed for cases with a count variable, cannot be applied. Therefore, the normal-LRT, developed to detect device signals among multiple devices, uses data from multiple sites/regions when the outcome of interest is a continuous variable.

Although the proposed LRT method based on normal model (Normal-LRT method) in this chapter is initiated by the motivation of multiple device performance comparison in terms of effectiveness, it may also be applied to safety surveillance, in situations where the safety events are derived from continuous measurements (e.g., hypoglycemia, an important safety endpoint for patients, is defined when the glucose level (continuous measurement) < 70 mg/dL). The continuous glucose level can also be explored among multiple devices in addition to the binary outcome (hypoglycemia). The major difference between other data mining methods (such as PRR, ROR, basic LRT) discussed in Chapter 2 and Chapter 3, and the proposed Normal-LRT method lies in the outcome variables (or the variable of interest). The Normal-LRT method deals with a continuous variable (that is assumed to be normally distributed), while the other methods consider a count variable.

9.2 Data Structure and Problem Formulation

9.2.1 Data structure

Suppose that a medical device study includes data from a total of S sites and I medical devices (of the same class). Let us fix a particular continuous variable such as weight, indexed by "j". Say, there are a total of $N_{i.s}$ subjects utilizing the device i in the site s, and each subject has an outcome measured on variable indexed by j. Ideally, $N_{i.s}$ individual-level measurements should be reported, i.e., $X_{ijs1}, X_{ijs2}, \cdots, X_{ijsN_{i.s}}$. While, in practice, the individual-level data may not be easily accessible, site-level summary data, such as sample mean $\bar{X}_{ijs} = \frac{\sum_{k=1}^{N_{i,s}} x_{ijsk}}{N_{i,s}}$, and the total number of subjects $N_{i.s}$, are often available for research purpose.

To clarify, an example of the site-level data structure is given in Table 9.4.

If the individual-level measurements, i.e., $X_{ijs1}, \cdots, X_{ijsk}, \cdots, X_{ijsN_{i.s}}$ are independent and normally distributed, with a device-specific mean and a common variance, i.e.,

$$X_{ijsk} \sim^{iid} N(\mu_{ij}, \sigma_j^2), k = 1, 2, \ldots, N_{i.s}.$$

Then, for site-level summary data presented in Table 9.4, we have

$$\bar{X}_{ijs} \sim^{iid} N(\mu_{ij}, \frac{\sigma_j^2}{N_{i.s}}), i = 1.., I, s = 1, \cdots, S,$$

where μ_{ij} is the mean of the variable of interest for device i. For fixed site s, one can collapse data from all other devices except i and calculate their sample mean $\bar{X}_{(-i)js} = \frac{\sum_{i' \neq i} N_{i'.s}\bar{X}_{i'js}}{\sum_{i' \neq i} N_{i'.s}}$. Letting v_{ij} denote the population mean of the variable for all other devices except device i, we have

$$\bar{X}_{(-i)js} \sim^{iid} N(v_{ij}, \sigma_j^2/(N_{..s} - N_{i.s})), i = 1, \cdots, I, s = 1, \cdots, S.$$

9.2.2 Problem formulation

The objective is to test the null hypothesis

$$H_0^j : \mu_{ij} = v_{ij} = \mu_{0j} \text{ for all devices } i, i = 1, 2, \ldots, I,$$

where the common mean μ_{0j} is unspecified, against the alternative hypothesis

$$H_a^j : \mu_{ij} > v_{ij} \text{for at least one device} i.$$

9.3 Normal-LRT method

9.3.1 MLRs of parameters μ_{ij}, v_{ij}, and σ_j^2

For fixed j, the likelihood function under the null hypothesis H_0^j is

$$L_0^j = L^j(\mu_{0j}) \propto \exp\left\{ -\frac{1}{2\hat{\sigma}_j^2} \sum_{i=1}^{I} \left[\sum_{s=1}^{S} N_{i.s}(\bar{X}_{ijs} - \mu_{0j})^2 \right.\right.$$
$$\left.\left. + \sum_{s=1}^{S} (N_{..s} - N_{i.s})(\bar{X}_{(-i)js} - \mu_{0j})^2 \right] \right\},$$

where $N_{..s} = \sum_{i=1}^{I} N_{i.s}$ denotes the total counts of utilization from all devices in site s. The likelihood function under alternative hypothesis is

$$L_a^j = L^j(\mu_{1j}, v_{1j}, \cdots, \mu_{Ij}, v_{Ij})$$

$$\propto \exp\left\{ -\frac{1}{(2\hat{\sigma}_j^2)} \sum_{i=1}^{I} \left[\sum_{s=1}^{S} N_{i.s}(\bar{X}_{ijs} - \mu_{ij})^2 + \sum_{s=1}^{S} (N_{..s} - N_{i.s})(\bar{X}_{(-i)js} - v_{ij})^2 \right] \right\}$$

.

It follows that the maximum likelihood estimate (MLE) of the parameter μ_{0j}, under H_0^j, is given by

$$\hat{\mu}_{0j} = \frac{\sum_{i=1}^{I}\left[\sum_{s=1}^{S} N_{i.s}\bar{X}_{ijs} + \sum_{s=1}^{S}(N_{..s} - N_{i.s})\bar{X}_{(-i)js}\right]}{\sum_{i=1}^{I}\left[\sum_{s=1}^{S} N_{i.s} + \sum_{s=1}^{S}(N_{..s} - N_{i.s})\right]} = \frac{X_{.j.}}{N_{...}},$$

and the MLEs of the parameters μ_{ij} and v_{ij}, under H_a^j, are given by

$$\hat{\mu}_{ij} = \frac{\sum_{s=1}^{S} N_{i.s}\bar{X}_{ijs}}{\sum_{s=1}^{S} N_{i.s}} = \frac{X_{ij.}}{N_{i..}},$$

$$\hat{v}_{ij} = \frac{\sum_{s=1}^{S}(N_{..s} - N_{i.s})\bar{X}_{(-i)js}}{\sum_{s=1}^{S}(N_{..s} - N_{i.s})} = \frac{X_{.j.}}{N_{...}} = \frac{X_{.j.} - X_{ij.}}{N_{...} - N_{i..}},$$

where $X_{ij.} = \sum_{s=1}^{S} N_{i.s}\bar{X}_{ijs}$ is the sum of measurements for j^{th} variable from i^{th} devices in all sites, $X_{.j.} = \sum_{i=1}^{I} X_{ij.}$ is the sum of measurements of jth variable from all devices in all sites, $N_{i..} = \sum_{s=1}^{S} N_{i.s}$ is the total counts of utilization of ith device in all sites, and $N_{...} = \sum_{i=1}^{I} N_{i..}$ is for all devices and all sites.

A commonly used strategy for estimating the nuisance parameter σ_j^2 is to use

$$\hat{\sigma}_j^2 = \frac{1}{IS}\sum_{i=1}^{I}\left[\sum_{s=1}^{S} N_{i.s}(\bar{X}_{ijs} - \hat{\mu}_{ij})^2\right],$$

and let it remain the same for both the null and alternative hypotheses.

9.3.2 Test statistic MLLR

With obtained parameter estimates, the likelihood ratio for a device i, is calculated as

$$\begin{aligned} LR_{ij} = \frac{L_a^{ij}}{L_0^{ij}} &= \frac{L^{ij}(\hat{\mu}_{ij}, \hat{v}_{ij})}{L^{ij}(\hat{\mu}_{0j})} \\ &= \exp\left\{-\frac{1}{2\hat{\sigma}_j^2}\left[\sum_{s=1}^{S} N_{i.s}[(\bar{X}_{ijs} - \hat{\mu}_{ij})^2 - (\bar{X}_{ijs} - \hat{\mu}_{0j})^2]\right.\right. \\ &\left.\left. + \sum_{s=1}^{S}(N_{..s} - N_{i.s})[(\bar{X}_{(-i)js} - \hat{v}_{ij})^2 - (\bar{X}_{(-i)js} - \hat{\mu}_{0j})^2]\right]\right\} \end{aligned}$$

and the log likelihood ratio for device i is

$$LLR_{ij} = log(LR_{ij}) = \frac{N_{i..}}{2\hat{\sigma}_j^2}(\hat{\mu}_{ij} - \hat{\mu}_{0j})(\hat{\mu}_{ij} - \hat{v}_{ij}).$$

Finally, the test statistic for testing H_0^j vs. H_a^j, is the maximum of the log likelihood ratio over all devices

$$MLLR_j = max_i\{LLR_{ij}I(\hat{\mu}_{ij} > \hat{v}_{ij})\},$$

where $I(.)$ is the indicator function.

Here, the methodology is formulated as a one-sided hypothesis test. To adapt it for two-sided test, the test statistic may be adjusted to $MLLR_j = max_i(LLR_{ij})$.

9.3.3 Permutation-based empirical distribution

Since the distribution of $MLLR_j$ under the null hypothesis is analytically intractable, permutation procedure is used [43] to construct the empirical distribution of $MLLR_j$ under the null hypothesis. Within each study site s, permutation is performed by randomly reallocating the observed data points among different devices (rows) for a fixed column s.

Under the null hypothesis, random permutation of data pair $(N_{i.s}, \bar{X}_{ijs})$ across rows is conducted column-wise for all sites to generate a new dataset, from which $MLLR_j$ is calculated. The purpose of permuting data column-wise, instead of globally (i.e., reallocating the observed data across the whole matrix), is to reduce the computational burden and to facilitate efficient generation of dataset under the null hypothesis. The above permutation process is repeated 1000 times and therefore a total of 1000 $MLLR_j$ values are calculated and used to construct the null distribution of $MLLR_j$.

Suppose the input data are structured as in Table 9.4, the column-wise permutation procedure to generate data under the null hypothesis is as follows:

- Step 1: For each site/column (i.e., the corresponding column variable) $s(s = 1, \cdots, S)$, randomly permute data in the I rows within that site. When permutation is finished for all S sites, a complete dataset is generated under null hypothesis. The value of $MLLR_j$ can be calculated from the generated dataset.

- Step 2: Repeat step 1 for $N_{sim} = 1000$ times to build the empirical distribution of $MLLR_j$.

Once the empirical distribution of $MLLR_j$ is established, a step-down process [80] is used to calculate p-values for signal detection . Briefly, the test statistic $MLLR_j$ based on observed dataset is compared against the upper $100(1-\alpha)$th percentile of the empirical $MLLR_j$ denoted as $MLLR_{j,\alpha}$. The null hypothesis is rejected if $MLLR_j \geq MLLR_{j,\alpha}$ and the associated device i with $LLR_{ij} = MLLR_j$ is considered the signal device. After that, one can step down to compare the $LLR_{i'j}$ from other devices against the cut-off value, i.e., $MLLR_{j,\alpha}$. Any device with a log likelihood value greater than the cutoff is identified as a signal. This step-down procedure theoretically controls the family-wise type-I error.

9.4 Application

For illustration, the proposed method is applied to a hypothetical case study following the real data pattern shown in studies for obesity treatment devices [28]. Note that there are 6 devices in this class for weight-loss treatment of patients with excessive fat accumulation that presents a risk to health [28]. Among the studies for these devices, the most commonly used endpoint for effectiveness is percent excess weight loss (%EWL) at a certain time point (e.g., 12 months), defined as (baseline weight - measured weight at the given time point)/(baseline weight - ideal body weight), where the ideal body weight is usually calculated as the weight corresponding to a body mass index (BMI) of $25kg/m^2$.

Assuming there is a post-market study or a registry collecting information about these 6 devices from a total of 15 regions, a description of the data generation process can be found in Appendix 9.7.1. Table 9.5 illustrates the structure of the example dataset. For device i and region s, $N_{i.s}$ is the number of patients who use device i in region s, and $\bar{X}_{ijs}$ is the mean %EWL for these patients. In this hypothetical dataset, devices 1 and 4 are used only in 8 regions, devices 2 and 5 are used only in 10 regions, whereas devices 3 and 6 are used in all 15 regions. The empty cells in Table 9.5 indicate that the device was not used in those sites (no patients in those cells), i.e., $N_{i.s} = 0$. Note that the cells with $N_{i.s} = 0$ do not have contribution to the likelihood function and permutation among non-empty cells. This effect of empty cells on model performance is evaluated through simulation (Appendix 9.7.2) and further discussed in the discussion section.

Given such a dataset (as shown in Table 9.5), the interest is to detect device signals that are associated with a significantly higher %EWL than other devices. We apply the proposed method to analyze the data and present the result in Table 9.6. We show that devices 1 and 5 are detected signals with significantly higher %EWL on average (the cutoff for LLR is 5.98 for the significance level 0.05), compared with that for other devices.

One thing to note is that this example is only used for illustration purposes (about how the proposed method can be used in real world applications where the data are collected from large post-market studies or registries), and the findings themselves should by no means be used to interpret the effectiveness of any device.

9.5 Simulation

9.5.1 Data simulation

A simulation study is conducted to evaluate performance of the normal-LRT method. Each setting is determined by 4 global parameters: # of sites (S), # of devices (I), # of true signal devices (T), and signal strength (δ). Under each setting, N_{sim} datasets are simulated via the following steps:

1. Let the mean be $\mu_{0j} + \delta \times \sigma_j$ for T signal devices, and μ_{0j} for the rest $I - T$ non-signal devices. (In the simulation, fix $\mu_{0j} = 0$ and $\sigma_j = 1$.)
2. Simulate the count $N_{i.s}$ from discrete uniform distribution $(3, 30), (30, 100)$, or $(100, 1000)$ to represent data with small, moderate, or large sample size respectively.
3. Simulate the data matrix $\bar{X}_{ijs}$ from multivariate normal distribution

$$(\bar{X}_{1j1}, \cdots, \bar{X}_{1jS}, \cdots, \bar{X}_{Ij1}, \cdots, \bar{X}_{IjS}) \sim$$

$$MultiN\left((\mu_{1j}\vec{1}^S, \cdots, \mu_{Ij}\vec{1}^S)_{1\times IS}, \sigma_j^2 \begin{bmatrix} \mathbf{N_1} & & \\ & \ddots & \\ & & \mathbf{N_I} \end{bmatrix}_{IS\times IS} \right)$$

where $\vec{1}^S = (1, \cdots, 1)_S$ is an all-ones vector in R^S, and $\mathbf{N_i}$ is a $S \times S$ diagonal matrix $diag(N_{i.1}^{-1}, N_{i.2}^{-1}, \cdots, N_{i.S}^{-1})$ for $i = 1, 2, \cdots, I$.

Based on N_{sim} datasets simulated via steps above, four metrics including the power, false discovery rate (FDR), sensitivity (ST), and type-I error rate (defined in Chapter 3), are calculated to evaluate performance of the normal-LRT method for detection of device signals.

9.5.2 Type-I error

In Table 9.7, 3 factors included to investigate the type-I error: (1) number of devices, (2) number of sites, (3) sample size $N_{i.s}$. Under each setting, $N_{sim} = 10000$. It shows that for all scenarios, the type-I error clusters around the desired alpha level (0.05) and therefore is well-controlled by the proposed method.

9.5.3 Power, sensitivity, and false discovery rate

The model performance is also investigated in terms of power, sensitivity (ST), and False Discovery Rate (FDR) in different settings. Under each setting,

N_{sim} = 1000. The results from selected scenarios are presented in Tables 9.8 to 9.10, where 3 factors, (1) number of devices, (2) number of sites, (3) number of signal devices, together with two other factors, mean difference δ and sample size $N_{i.s}$, are included to investigate the model performance. The effect of these factors on model performance is summarized below.

When the number of devices increases, with other parameters fixed, the power, sensitivity, and FDR fluctuate slightly but no clear trend is observed. For example, Table 9.8 shows that, with a moderate sample size $N_{i.s}$ (30, 100) and a small signal strength $\delta = 0.2$, as the number of devices increases from 3, 5, 10 to 15, the power fluctuates between 0.957 and 0.986; however, there is no clear increasing or decreasing trend.

The results also show that the method performs better with data from more sites. Table 9.9 shows that a higher number of sites corresponds to a higher power and sensitivity, and a lower FDR. For example, for a small sample size $N_{i.s}$ (3, 30) and a small signal strength $\delta = 0.2$, as the number of sites increases from 5 to 30, both power and sensitivity increase from about 20% to over 94%, and FDR declines from 6% to 0.1%.

Table 9.10 shows higher power values and lower FDR values for data with multiple signals compared to data with a single signal. As expected, enlarging the signal strength (the difference of the means, δ) or increasing the sample size ($N_{i.s}$) helps improve the model sensitivity and reduce the FDR (Tables 9.8 to 9.10). In summary, the normal-LRT approach controls FDR well, and maintains good sensitivity and power, especially when the signal strength $\delta \geq 0.5$.

9.6 Notes and Discussion

The proposed normal-LRT method incorporates the heterogeneity of continuous device-measures from varying sites using summary data combined from multiple sites and/or multiple studies. The site can be a typical site in a clinical trial study or a geographical region in any level (e.g., blocks, tracts, counties, states, countries, etc.).

The Normal-LRT method uses permutation [43] to obtain the empirical distribution of the test statistic under the null hypothesis, because simulating continuous data requires knowing the exact true distribution, including the true mean and variance, which are usually unknown in practice. On the other hand, assuming that the distributions of the outcome are homogeneous among different devices, permuting devices is a natural strategy to construct the null distribution of the test statistic, and thereby facilitates the identification of device signals with abnormal outcome values. It is worth noting that, in this method, column-wise permutation is used to serve as an alternative to whole matrix permutation to facilitate efficient null distribution construction, speed up the calculation of the p-values, and at the same time reduce computational memory requirement. This is because whole matrix permutation procedure can be time consuming especially when a large data matrix is involved, while perturbing data within each column (site) can be more efficient (under the null hypothesis that there is no difference among rows (devices)).

Through extensive simulation, the Normal-LRT method is shown to have reasonable power and sensitivity for device signal detection , with controlled type-I error. In addition, a hypothetical example with multiple obesity treatment devices from multiple sites is used to illustrate the application of the proposed method. Furthermore, this method can be applied in a variety of settings according to data availability and research interest, including but not limited to (1) searching for device signals using data from multiple sites (by letting the device be row variable, site be column variable), (2) searching for device signals using data including multiple looks for a fixed site (by letting the device be row variable, "look" (i.e., time point) be column variable), and (3) searching for site signals using data including multiple looks for a fixed device (by letting the site be row variable, "look" be column variable), etc.

In practice, the potential data sources for such applications include the data with multiple clinical trials for devices with similar indications, post-market approval studies including multiple devices, or registry data covering many regions. The number of regions/sites covered by the devices may not be the same for all the devices, resulting in missing cells in the data structured as in Table 9.4. Although the effect of empty cells does not affect the implementation of the model, its potential effect on model performance is evaluated through simulation (Appendix 9.7.2). The simulation indicates that a rate of empty cells above 50% may lead to the impeded performance (sensitivity lower than 60%), while the FDR is still under control. Note that permutation happens among non-empty cells. Particularly, in the extreme cases where most columns only have one or two non-empty cells, global permutation instead of column-wise permutation, should be applied to avoid biased construction of the null distribution.

The variances across different sites are assumed to be the same in the model. This assumption is a practical approach when the model is built upon a normal distribution with mean as the parameter of interest. The model can be extended to allow different variances among studies/sites. Another point to note is that, if the continuous outcome is extremely skewed, appropriate data pre-processing steps such as log transformation for variance stabilization, should be adopted to ensure the normality assumption.

TABLE 9.1
Description for hypothetical data.

	# of sites	range of $N_{i,s}$	range of X_{ijs}
Device 1	8	23-36	27.18-39.59
Device 2	10	12-25	12.54-31.99
Device 3	15	4-14	8.7-43.99
Device 4	8	7-16	11.82-24.14
Device 5	10	2-15	27.93-51.83
Device 6	15	8-14	3.49-38.44

9.7 Appendix

9.7.1 Data generation process for hypothetical case study

The hypothetical dataset used for application is generated based on the summary information on weight loss included in the safety and effectiveness reports of the 6 devices [28]. This dataset contains information regarding 6 obesity-treatment devices, with %EWL as the variable of interest. Table 9.1 lists the # of sites, the range of $N_{i.s}$ (# of patients who use device i in region s), and the range of $\bar{X}_{ijs}$ (mean %EWL at 12 months for patients who use device i in region s), by device. The standard deviation used to generate data for each cell is $\sigma = 26.35/N_{i.s}$.

9.7.2 Simulation for data including regions without data

The number of regions/sites covered by the devices may not be the same for all the devices. Therefore, a device may not have any data collected in some specific sites, resulting in empty cells in the data structured as in Table 9.4. Table 9.2 shows the parameter setup for a small simulation study conducted to explore the effect of empty cells on model performance. Table 9.2 shows the parameter setup.

For the signal device, the number of empty cells/sites are 8,5,2,0 corresponding to the proportion of empty cells as 80%, 50%, 20%, and 0% respectively. For all other devices combined, the proportion of empty cells is 0 or 50%. Table 9.3 presents the simulation results.

Table 9.3 also shows that a moderate percentage of empty cells ($< 20\%$) moderately influences sensitivity. However, a dataset with over 50% empty cells may lead to the impeded sensitivity ($< 60\%$). Overall, FDR is under 5% for all cases, which is desirable.

TABLE 9.2
Setup for missing data simulation.

Parameters	values
δ	0.5
$N_{i,s}$	(30, 100)
# of devices	5
# of sites	10
# of signal devices	1
% of empty cells for signal device	0, 20%, 50%, 80%
% of empty cells for all other devices combined	0, 50%

TABLE 9.3
Simulation results for data with empty cells, $N_{sim} = 1000$.

#(%) of empty cells for non-signal devices on average	#(%) of empty cells for signal devices	power	sensitivity	FDR
0 (0%)	0 (0%)	0.917	0.917	0
0 (0%)	2 (20%)	0.905	0.905	0
0 (0%)	5 (50%)	0.801	0.801	0
0 (0%)	8 (80%)	0.679	0.679	0
5 (50%)	0 (0%)	0.699	0.699	0
5 (50%)	2 (20%)	0.653	0.653	0
5 (50%)	5 (50%)	0.584	0.584	0
5 (50%)	8 (80%)	0.535	0.534	0

9.8 Tables and Figures

TABLE 9.4
Data matrix for I devices by S sites.

	Site 1	Site 2	⋯	Site s	⋯	Site S	Marginal
device 1	$N_{1.1}, \bar{X}_{1j1}$	$N_{1.2}, \bar{X}_{1j2}$	⋯	$N_{1.s}, \bar{X}_{1js}$	⋯	$N_{1.S}, \bar{X}_{1jS}$	$N_{1..}, \bar{X}_{1j.}$
device 2	$N_{2.1}, \bar{X}_{2j1}$	$N_{2.2}, \bar{X}_{2j2}$	⋯	$N_{2.s}, \bar{X}_{2js}$	⋯	$N_{2.S}, \bar{X}_{2jS}$	$N_{2..}, \bar{X}_{2j.}$
⋯	⋯	⋯	⋯	⋯	⋯	⋯	⋯
device i	$N_{i.1}, \bar{X}_{ij1}$	$N_{i.2}, \bar{X}_{ij2}$	⋯	$N_{i.s}, \bar{X}_{ijs}$	⋯	$N_{i.S}, \bar{X}_{ijS}$	$N_{i..}, \bar{X}_{ij.}$
⋯	⋯	⋯	⋯	⋯	⋯	⋯	⋯
device I	$N_{I.1}, \bar{X}_{Ij1}$	$N_{I.2}, \bar{X}_{Ij2}$	⋯	$N_{I.s}, \bar{X}_{Ijs}$	⋯	$N_{I.S}, \bar{X}_{IjS}$	$N_{I..}, \bar{X}_{Ij.}$
Marginal	$N_{..1}, \bar{X}_{.j1}$	$N_{..2}, \bar{X}_{.j2}$	⋯	$N_{..s}, \bar{X}_{.js}$	⋯	$N_{..S}, \bar{X}_{.jS}$	$N_{...}, \bar{X}_{.j.}$

TABLE 9.5
Example dataset for the case study, $(N_{i.s}, \bar{X}_{ijs})$.

	region1	region2	region3-7	region8	region9	region10	region11-14	region15
device 1	(23, 37.7)	(34, 36.1)	⋯	(36, 36.3)	no data	no data	no data	no data
device 2	(25, 28.5)	(14, 25.6)	⋯	(14, 22.3)	(18, 32.0)	(12, 23.9)	no data	no data
device 3	(7, 25.4)	(10, 44.0)	⋯	(7, 8.7)	(10, 23.9)	(8, 28.3)	⋯	(11, 35.4)
device 4	(12, 23.8)	(10, 18.9)	⋯	(15, 18.1)	no data	no data	no data	no data
device 5	(9, 44.4)	(2, 30.4)	⋯	(8, 39.9)	(6, 28.8)	(5, 51.8)	no data	no data
device 6	(12, 13.5)	(11, 20.9)	⋯	(11, 14.0)	(14, 15.6)	(11, 23.4)	⋯	(13, 22.8)

TABLE 9.6
Analysis result for the case study.

Device	$\hat{\mu}_i$	$\hat{v}_i$	LLR_i	p-value
Device 1	35.39	25.42	13.75	0
Device 2	22.7	29.4	0	1
Device 3	29.63	27.87	0.27	0.986
Device 4	19.37	29.11	0	1
Device 5	38.23	27.06	7.55	0.021
Device 6	21.74	29.69	0	1

TABLE 9.7
Type-I error ($N_{sim} = 10000$).

# of devices	$N_{i,s}$ range	# of sites			
		5	10	20	30
3	(3, 30)	0.056	0.053	0.049	0.054
3	(30, 100)	0.057	0.054	0.045	0.053
3	(100, 1000)	0.056	0.055	0.052	0.051
5	(3, 30)	0.049	0.047	0.048	0.05
5	(30, 100)	0.047	0.05	0.048	0.052
5	(100, 1000)	0.045	0.052	0.049	0.048
10	(3, 30)	0.05	0.047	0.05	0.052
10	(30, 100)	0.048	0.046	0.048	0.054
10	(100, 1000)	0.048	0.052	0.051	0.05
15	(3, 30)	0.05	0.046	0.054	0.055
15	(30, 100)	0.051	0.048	0.05	0.056
15	(100, 1000)	0.053	0.053	0.054	0.05

TABLE 9.8
Effect of number of devices, $N_{sim} = 1000$ (fix number of sites = 10, number of signals =1).

$N_{i,s}$	# of	power vs. δ			sensitivity vs. δ			FDR vs. δ		
	devices	0.2	0.5	2	0.2	0.5	2	0.2	0.5	2
(3, 30)	3	0.419	0.991	1	0.418	0.991	1	0.002	0	0
(3, 30)	5	0.418	0.997	1	0.414	0.997	1	0.01	0	0
(3, 30)	10	0.432	1	1	0.425	1	1	0.017	0	0
(3, 30)	15	0.4	1	1	0.383	1	1	0.048	0.001	0
(30, 100)	3	0.957	1	1	0.957	1	1	0	0	0
(30, 100)	5	0.978	1	1	0.978	1	1	0	0	0
(30, 100)	10	0.986	1	1	0.986	1	1	0.003	0	0
(30, 100)	15	0.977	1	1	0.977	1	1	0.003	0	0
(100, 1000)	3	1	1	1	1	1	1	0	0	0
(100, 1000)	5	1	1	1	1	1	1	0	0	0
(100, 1000)	10	1	1	1	1	1	1	0	0	0
(100, 1000)	15	1	1	1	1	1	1	0	0	0

TABLE 9.9
Effect of number of sites, $N_{sim} = 1000$ (fix number of devices = 5, number of signals =1).

$N_{i,s}$	# of	power vs. δ			sensitivity vs. δ			FDR vs. δ		
	devices	0.2	0.5	2	0.2	0.5	2	0.2	0.5	2
(3, 30)	5	0.193	0.867	1	0.181	0.867	1	0.062	0	0
(3, 30)	10	0.418	0.997	1	0.414	0.997	1	0.01	0	0
(3, 30)	20	0.825	1	1	0.825	1	1	0	0	0
(3, 30)	30	0.942	1	1	0.942	1	1	0.001	0	0
(30, 100)	5	0.702	1	1	0.701	1	1	0.001	0	0
(30, 100)	10	0.978	1	1	0.978	1	1	0	0	0
(30, 100)	20	1	1	1	1	1	1	0	0	0
(30, 100)	30	1	1	1	1	1	1	0	0	0
(100, 1000)	5	1	1	1	1	1	1	0	0	0
(100, 1000)	10	1	1	1	1	1	1	0	0	0
(100, 1000)	20	1	1	1	1	1	1	0	0	0
(100, 1000)	30	1	1	1	1	1	1	0	0	0

TABLE 9.10
Effect of number of signals, $N_{sim} = 1000$ (fix number of devices = 15, number of sites = 5).

$N_{i,s}$	# of devices	power vs. δ 0.2	0.5	2	sensitivity vs. δ 0.2	0.5	2	FDR vs. δ 0.2	0.5	2
(3, 30)	1	0.17	0.902	1	0.149	0.901	1	0.126	0.002	0
(3, 30)	2	0.221	0.958	1	0.108	0.683	1	0.048	0	0
(3, 30)	3	0.239	0.943	1	0.082	0.469	1	0.015	0	0
(30, 100)	1	0.748	1	1	0.743	1	1	0.009	0	0
(30, 100)	2	0.815	1	1	0.509	0.995	1	0.004	0	0
(30, 100)	3	0.823	1	1	0.35	0.904	1	0	0	0
(100, 1000)	1	1	1	1	1	1	1	0	0	0
(100, 1000)	2	1	1	1	0.982	0.997	1	0	0	0
(100, 1000)	3	1	1	1	0.868	0.965	1	0	0	0

10

Use of LRT in Site Selection

10.1 Background

This chapter describes the LRT method and application in site selection for inspections ([142]). The U.S. Food and Drug Administration (FDA) conducts on-site inspections and data audits through Bioresearch Monitoring (BIMO) [46] program to assure the quality and integrity of data submitted to the agency in the pre-approval and post-approval processes. The BIMO program was established in 1977 by a task force which included representatives from the drug, biologics, medical device, veterinary medicine, and food sectors. It provides regulatory oversight of clinical investigators, nonclinical laboratories (animal studies), sponsors, monitors, contract research organizations, and institutional review boards in support of the pre-market and post-market review program. It not only provides protection of the rights and welfare of the thousands of human subjects and animals involved in FDA regulated studies but also has become a cornerstone in support of new product approval and market applications.

The complexity of clinical studies across multiple sites poses challenges to both the companies and FDA for selecting sites for inspection. For example, sponsors/investigators conducting clinical studies in multiple sites face significant management challenges to maintain data quality and integrity, while obtaining and retaining an adequate sample within targeted populations [54]. Since not all the clinical sites and investigators have the same training and experience in coordinating clinical studies across multiple study sites, the variability in trial management such as protocol implementation, data collection, and data reporting, could pose sizeable challenges to the companies and investigators. The patient-level variability across sites can also present a challenge to determine which sites should be considered for inspection.

Investigators select sites for inspection by looking at factors of interest, such as the efficacy and safety information, site inspection history, patient characteristics, and site enrollment. For instance, an extremely high success rate of efficacy in a site may indicate suspicious data fraud issues, protocol deviations may be an indicator for investigating the integrity of trial conduct. However, these methods are ad-hoc, based on descriptive statistics, and lack sound statistical rigors. In addition, site selection involves many sites and variables, making it difficult to select sites using manual check. Therefore, statistical tools are needed to help in selecting aberrant sites.

The proposed technical framework includes construction of a p-value matrix obtained by applying statistical tests to each variable, and two novel statistical approaches: Fisher combination approach, and likelihood ratio test (LRT) approach, to integrate information from the p-value matrix. The proposed approaches produce combined p-value scores and rankings of the sites; and the sites that have small combined p-values are ranked high, henceforth referred to as site signals, and may be selected for inspection.

The proposed approaches are applied to a hypothetical dataset reflecting the real data pattern observed in one CDRH premarket approval (PMA) submission for a diagnostic device. A series of simulations are used to investigate the accuracy of the methods identifying the correct site signals, the type-I error, and false discovery rates. The method discussed here is used in CDRH BIMO site selection. Related work for identifying location differences between each center and all other centers in monitoring clinical trial data gathered across centers is discussed in Ref. [37].

10.2 Data and P-value Matrix

We consider a clinical study that consists of I study sites with subjects enrolled in the ith site. The collected dataset from all subjects includes information on variables of interest to the investigators, such as age, BMI, protocol deviation, serious adverse events (AEs), non-serious adverse events, etc.

Using the aforementioned dataset, one can construct a p-value matrix, by following Steps 1 and 2.

- Step 1: Conduct statistical tests for each variable and generate p-values by site. We first apply appropriate statistical tests to each variable to evaluate whether a site is different from all other sites combined, and that generates the p-value for each site. For a given variable, this provides preliminary information on whether each individual site is different from the other sites combined. The LRT method [80, 81] is used for count variables and random effects model [34, 37] for continuous variables for generating the p-value by site for individual variables (Appendix 10.7.1).

- Step 2: Construction of p-value matrix for overall assessment after statistical tests have been conducted for each variable in step 1, the resulting p-values are organized in an $I \times J$ matrix as shown in Table 10.4. Note that the total number of sites I and the total number of variables J can vary from single digit number to hundreds of thousands.

To select sites for inspection, one needs to integrate the information on p-values from all the variables/tests in the matrix, instead of looking at each variable/test separately. In Section 10.3, we propose two novel approaches to provide site ranking by integrating all information from all variables/tests.

10.3 Statistical Approaches for Site Ranking Generation from P-value Matrix

For each site/row, the p-values from all columns/tests are combined to form a p-value score (single score) for that site. The aim is to rank the sites utilizing the combined p-value scores and then to select the "top sites" for inspection. Here, we propose two methods for generating the combined p-value score for each site: Fisher combination approach, and LRT approach. Note that we use the words "column", "test", and "variable" interchangeably in the rest of the chapter.

10.3.1 Fisher combination approach

The Fisher combination approach proposed here is a site ranking approach using Fisher's method [47], which is a technique to combine the p-values from several statistical tests. The assumption that all p_{ij} are independent is reasonable because different sites are independent and even for correlated variables. whether that correlation transfers into p-values is not known. For each variable, under the null hypothesis that the variable effect for a site is the same as the remaining sites, $p_{ij} \sim^{iid} U[0,1]$. Then, the log transformed p-values $-2log(p_{ij}) \sim^{iid} \chi^2_2$, i.e., a Chi-squared distribution with 2 degrees of freedom according to Fisher's method [47]. For a fixed site i, all statistical tests can be combined across all J columns in row i as, $s_i = \sum_{j=1}^{J} -2log(p_{ij}) \sim \chi^2_{2J}$, a Chi-squared distribution with $2J$ degrees of freedom; and all statistical tests for other sites, except the values in row i, can be summed up over the whole matrix as $s_{-i} = \sum_{i' \neq i} s_{i'} \sim \chi^2_{2J(I-1)}$, a Chi-squared distribution with $2J(I-1)$ degrees of freedom. Note that for p-value=0, the corresponding log transformation gives a value of infinity. To avoid this problem, and also to reduce the influence from extremely small p-values, any p-value $< 1e-10$ is set to $1e-10$.

With calculated s_i and s_{-i} for each site i, we further calculate the p-values under their Chi-squared distributions, namely $\tilde{p}_i = P(\chi^2_{2J} < s_i)$ and $\tilde{p}_{-i} = P(\chi^2_{2J(I-1)} > s_{-i})$. If i^{th} site is distinct from other sites, the tail probability $\tilde{p}_i = P(\chi^2_{2J} > s_i)$ should be small and $PR_i = \frac{\tilde{p}_{-i}}{\tilde{p}_i}$ for $i = 1, \cdots, I$ will be large. If the sites are similar, PR_i should be the same among all sites. Therefore, we would like to consider null hypothesis $H_0 : PR_1 = PR_i = \cdots =$

PR_0, with PR_0 unknown, against the alternative hypothesis H_a : at least one $PR_i > PR_0$. The test statistic is then defined as $MRR = max_i(PR_i)$ over all sites.

Since the distribution of MRR under null is analytically not tractable, a bootstrap resampling method is applied to obtain its empirical null distribution. For each column j, new p_{ij} values for all sites are sampled from the original p-values in column j in the observed data with replacement, assuming that the p_{ij} values in one column is exchangeable and the sites are not different. The resampling process is repeated for all columns. After one resampling process, a new p-value matrix is created and a test statistic MPR denoted as MPR_b is calculated accordingly. The above process is repeated for B times ($B > 10,000$) to construct the empirical distribution of MPR assuming no difference among sites and PR_i values same for all sites. Finally, the p-value score against H_0 is calculated as $\frac{1}{B}\sum_{b=1}^{B} I(MPR_b \geq MPR_{obs})$, where MPR_{obs} is obtained from the observed data. If H_0 is rejected, i.e., p-value < 0.05, the site corresponding to MPR_{obs} has different PR value compared with other sites and thus may be identified as a site signal (strongest). With observed PR_i , p-value score for each site i is calculated as $\frac{1}{B}\sum_{b=1}^{B} I(MPR_b \geq PR_i)$, the calculated p-values (smallest to largest) can be used to rank the sites in descending order, and the sites with p-value < 0.05 are additional possible site signals.

10.3.2 LRT approach

Given a matrix of p-values, with each entry on the continuous scale in $[0, 1]$, we transform the p-values in the matrix, with entries, as binary values "0" or "1", using a pre-specified threshold value ($thred$). For example, if $thred = 0.1$, a cell entry is assigned a value "1" when its p-value< 0.1 (this test/variable is a "significant test/variable"), and a value "0" otherwise. Table 10.5 provides an example of dichotomized p-value matrix with $thred = 0.1$. The resulting dichotomized matrix can be further summarized as a count table (Table 10.6), and can be analyzed as defined below.

$$
\begin{aligned}
c_{ij} &= 1 \text{ if } 0 \leq p_{ij} < 0.1 \\
&= 0 \text{ if } p_{ij} \geq 1 \text{ when } thred = 0.1 \\
&NA \text{ otherwise.}
\end{aligned}
$$

We assume that $n_i \sim^{ind} Pois(P_i p_i)$ and $(n. - n_i) \sim^{ind} Pois((P - P_i)p_{-i})$ for all sites $i = 1, ..., I$, where p_i is the rate of "significant variables/tests" with $p_{ij} < thred$ for site i and p_{-i} is the rate of "significant tests/variables" for all the other sites except site i. We would like to consider the null hypothesis that $H_0 : p_i = p_{-i} = p_0$ for all $i = 1, \cdots, I$ against the alternative hypothesis $H_a : p_i > p_{-i}$ for at least one i. Under the null hypothesis, all the sites are similar. We can now apply the LRT method described in Chapter 3, to test if a site has a higher rate of "significant variable/test" than the other sites (Appendix 10.7.1, Test based on LRT for count variables).

Finally, the test p-value scores are used to rank the sites in descending order such that top ranked sites can be selected for inspection. Note that before applying the LRT method, an extra parameter, *thred*, needs to be pre-specified whose value can affect the site ranking.

10.4 Application to a Case Study

We illustrate the use of two site ranking approaches by applying them to a hypothetical case study reflecting the real data pattern observed in one CDRH premarket approval (PMA) submission for a diagnostic device. Of the 16 sites in this PMA, each site has different number of subjects ranging from tens to hundreds. The original dataset includes subject-level binary variables such as serious adverse event (SAE), protocol deviation, and continuous variables such as blood pressure, BMI, etc. Appropriate statistical tests (i.e., basic LRT for count variable (discussed in Chapter 3) and random effects model for continuous variable (presented in Appendix 10.7.1)) are performed for each variable, with each test reporting a per-site p-value denoting if a site is different from other sites for a certain variable. For illustration purpose, we present Table 10.7 as part of the constructed p-value matrix from 20 statistical variables/tests. In practice, the p-value matrix can contain tens to hundreds of statistical variables/tests. Note that we use the columns as Var1,..., Var20, to represent statistical test results for different variables of interest. For example, Var1 (percentage of subjects with protocol deviation) may suggest that patients in sites 5,7,13 have significantly higher rate of protocol deviation than patients in other sites. The goal here is to summarize the information in the p-value matrix and provide a p-value score for each site to represent its atypical property when compared with other sites. Therefore, both the LRT and Fisher combination approaches are utilized to analyze the matrix and the resulting per-site p-value scores are shown in the last two columns of Table 10.7.

Results from both methods indicate that Site 7 is significantly different from other sites. Considering that there are a small number of variables/tests in the data, together with the fact that usually top 3 sites are selected for investigation, we rank the p-values and extract the top 3 sites from either method. The LRT method suggests Sites 7, 13, and 3, whereas the Fisher combination method suggests Sites 7, 13, and 8 as the top sites. Both the LRT and Fisher methods agree with each other for the top 2 sites but recommend different sites for the top 3rd one (LRT method indicates Site 3 and Fisher combination method indicates Site 8 as the top 3rd). Evaluation of the complete p-value matrix indicates that the difference can be explained by Site 3 having more significant variables (at the pre-specified *thred*) than Site 8 which has only one significant variable at a high significance level (p-value$<$ 0.001). LRT method takes into account only the number of significant (at the chosen thred) tests whereas Fisher combination method takes into account the extent of significance of a p-value in the p-value matrix.

10.5 Comprehensive Simulation Study

Next we perform extensive simulations to evaluate the performance of the two proposed approaches to combine the p-values by site and generate the rankings of the sites. The parameters considered in the simulation and the steps are shown below.

1. Define global parameter setting: number of sites (rows), number of tests/variables for each site (column).
2. Generate the dataset (p-value matrix data) from uniform distribution, i.e., for each cell (i^{th} site and jth test) in the p-value matrix, simulate $p_{ij} \sim U[0,1]$. This dataset can be considered as generated under the global null hypothesis (that corresponds to the p-values being distributed homogenously among sites for each variable). The type-I error can be evaluated using this data.
3. Consider the following signal parameter setting: number of site signals, number of significant variables/tests for each site signal and the significance level (stronger with smaller p_{ij} values) for each variable/test to evaluate other performance characteristics (like power and sensitivity) of the proposed approaches.
4. Generate p-values for the significant variables/tests within each site signal (Appendix 10.7.2).

10.5.1 Performance characteristics

The model performance can be evaluated in terms of type-I error, pseudo-sensitivity, sensitivity, specificity and False discovery rate (FDR) defined below. N_{sim} is the total number of simulations.

1. For data simulated from global null,

$$\text{type-I error} = \frac{\text{\#of times rejecting the global null hypothesis}}{N_{sim}}$$

2. For data simulated with at least one site signal,

$$Sensitivity = \frac{1}{N_{sim}} \sum_{i=1}^{I=N_{sim}} \frac{\text{\#of true signals detected in the } l^{th}\text{simulated data}}{\text{total\#of true signals in the } l^{th}\text{simulated data}}$$

$$Specificity = \frac{1}{N_{sim}} \sum_{i=1}^{I=N_{sim}} \frac{\text{\#of true non-signals identified in the } l^{th}\text{simulated data}}{\text{total\#of non-signals in the } l^{th}\text{simulated data}}$$

$$FDR = \frac{1}{N_{sim}} \sum_{i=1}^{I=N_{sim}} \frac{\text{\#of signals falsely detected in the } l^{th}\text{simulated data}}{\text{total\#of detected signals in the } l^{th}\text{simulated data}}$$

Usually, due to limited resources, top sites (for example, 3 or 5) with relatively smaller per-site p-value scores among all sites, are extracted for site inspection. Note that a site with a p-value of 0.1 or higher may also be selected for inspection if the ranking of the site is high among all sites. To understand the site selection performance using ranking criteria, we propose another performance characteristic, termed here as pseudo-sensitivity. Suppose there are k true site signals in the data, after analysis by LRT or Fisher combination ranking approach, sites are ranked by per-site p-value scores and the top k sites are extracted, then,

$$\text{pseudo-sensitivity} = \text{\#of true signals within the top ranked } \ k \text{ sites}/k.$$

If pseudo-sensitivity is high but the sensitivity is low, the used approach (LRT or Fisher combination approach) can still provide good site ranking but may not be sensitive enough to claim a top ranked site as "statistically significant".

10.5.2 Results

- Type-I error

  The p-value matrix is constructed by values generated from $U[0,1]$ without any site signals. Each simulated dataset, i.e., simulated p-value matrix, is analyzed by both LRT and Fisher combination ranking approaches. Table 10.8 shows the simulation settings for different experimental conditions. Ten thousand simulations are performed under each experimental scenario, and the type-I error is calculated by the number of times the global null hypothesis is rejected (i.e., at least one per-site p-value score < 0.05) divided by the total number of simulations, e.g., 10,000.

  Two factors, # of sites (i.e., the total number of rows I in the original $I \times J$ matrix) and # of tests for each site (i.e., the total number of columns J

in the original $I \times J$ matrix) are investigated for influence on type-I error. Table 10.9 shows the type-I errors of LRT approach and Fisher combination approach. In sum, for all scenarios, the type-I error with the LRT approach is much smaller than the pre-specified level of significance ($\alpha = 0.05$), making that approach conservative. On the other hand, the Fisher combination approach has a slightly inflated type-I error, probably because p-values from $U[0,1]$ distribution are directly employed for modeling without column-wise adjustment for multiple testing. Although not shown here, simulated dataset with each test/column adjusted by "Benjamini Hochberg (BH)" [23] method beforehand and then analyzed by Fisher combination approach show that the Fisher combination approach controls type-I error.

- Multiple signals for sensitivity, specificity and FDR

  To have a comprehensive understanding of the model behavior, four important factors including (1) # of sites, (2) # of tests for each site, (3) percentage of significant tests within the site signal, and (4) the significance level of each test (i.e., the magnitude of p-values for significant tests), are investigated separately in terms of sensitivity (and pseudo-sensitivity), specificity, and FDR. One additional important factor, i.e., the total number of site signals in the data, is examined along with these four factors. The default settings for the simulations are indicated in Table 10.10, and the corresponding results are in Tables 10.11–10.14. For example, to check the effect of total # of sites I (Table 10.11), we change only the number of sites from 10 to 100 while keeping all the other parameters at default values.

  Tables 10.11–10.14 show that both methods have high specificity and controlled FDR. In addition, the Fisher combination method has higher sensitivity than the LRT method. However, the pseudo-sensitivities are reasonable for both methods (almost all results have pseudo-sensitivity>0.5).

  Table 10.11 indicates that given a fixed percentage of site signals (e.g., 5%, 10%, or 20%), increasing the number of total sites, I, will mildly decrease the sensitivity.

  As shown in Table 10.12, when the number of tests per site, J, is increased, the sensitivity of both methods increases.

  Table 10.13 shows the effect of number of significant tests per site signal when there are a total of 50 tests (i.e., $J = 50$). When the percentage of significant tests among all tests increases, the sensitivity of both methods increases.

  Table 10.14 shows the effect of significance level of individual test/column. P-values for each significant test were simulated from $U[0, 0.05)$, $U[0, 0.025)$, and $U[0, 0.01)$ for scenarios of mild, moderate, and high significance levels, respectively. As expected, the LRT method is not affected because the dichotomization process of LRT approach diminishes the influence of the magnitude of p-values given $thred = 0.1$. The Fisher combination method is highly influenced by the significance level. With higher significance level, e.g., 0.01, the Fisher combination can gain higher sensitivity. Both methods can retain adequate pseudo-sensitivity, specificity, and FDR under all the three significance levels (mild, moderate, and high).

10.6 Notes and Discussion

The proposed site ranking framework for selecting study sites includes two stages (Stage-I: tests for individual variables/tests and p-value matrix generation; and Stage-II: integrating the information from the p-value matrix using the LRT and Fisher combination approaches, and obtaining the site rankings). The approaches provide support in the site selection process, and output reports for easy interpretation. To determine which sites are selected for inspection, the BIMO reviewers consider the outputs from the statistical approaches discussed here along with factors such as site size, inspection history, case report forms, etc. Note that it is important to include all variables of interest for the p-value matrix generation, as they may affect the site rankings and missing important variables can potentially introduce bias in the performance of the proposed methods in finding the sites for inspection. However, with the help of the proposed statistical approach, the investigators only need to input the variables/factors of interest. The statistical methods will perform the analysis for each variable and, with all the variables combined, output each site's overall ranking. Therefore, the proposed statistical approaches can improve the investigators' work efficiency and help them make less biased decision, and ultimately reduce the cost of site-selection.

Through extensive simulation work, we have shown that the proposed site ranking approaches can detect site signals, with varying performance depending on several important factors. The type-I errors and FDRs are all well controlled for both methods. The sensitivity of Fisher combination method is higher than LRT method since LRT method uses the dichotomized data in the p-value matrix whereas the Fisher combination method uses all information. With a large number of variables included in the p-value matrix, higher sensitivity can be achieved for both methods (for example, sensitivity > 0.6 to 0.7). Both the methods have good specificity and controlled $FDR < 0.05$. Even though the sensitivity may not always be high (< 0.6) for some generated datasets (with smaller site sizes, and fewer number of variables), both the approaches have adequate accuracy (pseudo-sensitivity > 0.9) in finding the top site signals for inspection. This is reasonable since usually one can only inspect a small number of study sites due to limited resources, and the selection of most suspect sites with low false discovery rate is important.

Furthermore, in medical device clinical studies, the total sample sizes are determined for the overall study evaluation, instead of for each site evaluation. For small sample size (i.e., site size between 1 and 20 subjects), there may not be enough power to detect significant sites for each test/column in the individual variable evaluation step (Stage-I). As a result, the p-value matrix may have small percentage of tests with small p-values (i.e. $p < 0.05$). However, as the order of the ranking is correct one can still select the sites with top rankings (even for larger than 0.05 or 0.1 p-value scores). For medical device clinical studies with many small sites, 3–5 sites with top rankings may be selected first; the selected sites can then be further evaluated for each variable with respect to the magnitude of the observed site difference. Clinical input is required to support the final decision on site selection and to determine whether the observed difference is clinically meaningful.

In addition to the small sample size, missing data may also influence the result in the individual variable evaluation step (Stage-I). In site selection, the unbalance of percent missing data among sites is also an important factor that can be treated as an additional count variable. Then the resulting p-value matrix, augmented with the p-values from testing for missing information, could potentially help generate improved sensitivity by both approaches.

Although both the Fisher combination and LRT approaches have high specificity, the sensitivity of the Fisher combination approach is higher than that of the LRT approach, because of retention of magnitude of p-value matrix entries. However, LRT approach, which depends on the binary transformation of the p-value matrix, can potentially accommodate information not given as a p-value matrix. For example, a set of clinically meaningful criteria is set up for the variables of interest. Based on the criteria for each variable (column), a site is denoted as "1" if it does not meet the requirement of that variable, and "0" otherwise. Following this process for all the other variables, a binary matrix, instead of a p-value matrix, can be constructed. By counting the number of "1"s (the number of variables for which a site is an outlier) and the number of "0"s (the number of variables for which a site is an inlier), the proposed LRT approach, which is designed for the count data, can naturally be applied for each site.

Instead of applying LRT or random effects model (Appendix 10.7.1) to generate p-values at Satge-I, adding appropriate statistical tests for a single variable to create a p-value matrix with more columns may improve the sensitivity of both approaches. Specifically, one can add columns of additional tests [77] for categorical (or ordinal) variables, such as Proportional Reporting Ratios [45], Chi-square test methods [61], Beta-Binomial model [36]. Similarly, one can also add columns of additional tests for continuous variables, such as tests for variance/standard deviation. This may result in an improved sensitivity of the proposed approaches at the site-ranking step (Stage-II).

If a sponsor/investigator is interested in the real-time monitoring of the study sites, the proposed approaches can be adapted for interim analysis. If the study is monitored over a period of time and multiple looks (K) are scheduled, the control of overall type-I error across all looks needs to be attained, for example, by an alpha spending function. Then, at a certain look k, the dataset including data up to date with variables of interests are analyzed by the proposed approaches. The calculated per-site p-value score is compared against the pre-set alpha level at look k. If the comparison shows that a specific site is significantly different from other sites at an interim look, the sponsor/investigator can immediately conduct field inspection for that site and reveal/solve problems in a timely manner. Since problematic sites can be identified during an early phase of the study and appropriate adjustment can be made well ahead of the submission to the regulatory agencies, the total cost of the clinical studies may be reduced considerably by applying the proposed approaches.

We note that both the LRT and the Fisher combination approach assume independence among tests/columns when obtaining the final ranking scores from the p-value matrix. However, in case of several tests applied to the same variable, tests may be correlated, resulting in correlated p-values in the matrix. Methods have been developed to approximate the distribution of combined correlated p-values [92] and their accuracy is evaluated by Alves et al. [19, 92] To understand the impact of correlation, the Fisher combination approach is extended to allow for correlation among p-values (details in Appendix 10.7.3) and the simulation shows that the extended Fisher combination approach with correlation adjustment is generally more conservative in terms of the final p-value scores than its original version without correlation adjustment. Both Fisher combination approaches with and without correlation adjustment share similar pseudo-sensitivities, suggesting that both approaches have comparable performances in terms of the accuracy of site rankings.

The BIMO LRT inspection Statistical Software (BLISS) is developed based on the LRT approach and Fisher combination approach to identify sites as signals that are different compared to other sites in a clinical trial. BLISS provides an interactive interface, including data loading, variable selection, parameter option, and final report (ranking tables plus visualization). BLISS was programmed using R and JavaScript and was displayed using Shiny dashboard by RStudio. The combination of R and JavaScript offers the freedom to generate more dynamic and interactive features in both the back-end and the front-end. These dynamic features offer end users more flexibilities to understand and analyze site selection data. This tool is currently used to provide information for supporting the inspection site selection during BIMO review in FDA Center for Devices and Radiological Health (CDRH).

10.7 Appendix

10.7.1 Statistical tests for individual variables

Given a dataset with variables from all sites, the first step is to conduct appropriate statistical tests, for each variable, to check if any site is different from the others. Here, we focus on two statistical models, namely LRT and random effects model, for count and continuous variables, respectively.

- Test based on LRT for count variables

  For a binary variable denoting whether a patient may have a serious adverse event (SAE), a non-serious adverse event (NSAE), a protocol deviation, or death, data from all subjects within a site can be summarized by a count variable (Var_j) as shown in Table 10.1, where the first column represents the site ID, the second column represents the number of patients with at least one event for Var_j , in each of the sites, and the third column represents the total number of patients in the corresponding site.

TABLE 10.1
Data structure for a count variable.

Site ID	# of patients for Var_j	Total # of patients
1	n_{1j}	$n_{1.}$
...	...	...
i	n_{ij}	$n_{i.}$
...	...	...
I	n_{Ij}	$n_{I.}$
Total	$n_{.j}$	$n_{..}$

With data described in the above count table, the likelihood ratio test (LRT) method described in Chapter 3 can be applied to identify the sites that are different from the other sites for Var_j.

We assume that $n_{ij} \sim^{ind} Pois(n_{i.}p_{ij})$, and $n_{.j} - n_{ij} \sim^{ind} Pois(n_{..} - n_{i.})q_{ij})$ for all sites $i = 1, \cdots, I$, where p_{ij} is the parameter representing the risk/rate of site o for Var_j and q_{ij} is the parameter representing the risk/rate of all the other sites combined, except site i. The likelihood ratio for site i, fixed at column j (Var_j), is

$$LR_{ij} = \frac{L_{H_a}}{L_{H_0}} = \frac{(\hat{p}_{ij})^{n_{ij}}(\hat{q}_{ij})^{n_{.j}-n_{ij}}}{(\hat{p}_0)^{n_{.j}}} = \frac{(\frac{n_{ij}}{n_{i.}})^{n_{ij}}(\frac{n_{.j}-n_{ij}}{n_{..}-n_{i.}})^{n_{.j}-n_{ij}}}{(\frac{n_{.j}}{n_{..}})^{n_{.j}}}$$

and the log likelihood ratio is $LLR_{ij} = n_{ij}log(\hat{p}_{ij}) + (n_{.j} - n_{ij})log(\hat{q}_{ij}) - n_{.j}log(\hat{p}_0)$.

The test statistic for testing $H_0 : p_{ij} = q_{ij} = p_0$ versus $H_a : p_{ij} > q_{ij}$is the maximum log likelihood ratio ($MLLR_j$) across all sites $i = 1, \cdots, I$, where $\hat{p}_{ij} > \hat{p}_{ij}$, i.e. $MLLR_j = max_i(LLR_i)I(\hat{p}_{ij} > \hat{q}_{ij})$. An empirical distribution of $MLLR_j$ can be obtained from the data generated using Monte Carlo (MC) simulation assuming $H_0 : p_i = q_i$ for all $i = 1, \cdots, I$. The p-value score for each site can also be determined by ranking the observed LLR_j in the empirical distribution of $MLLR_j$. The sites with p-values < 0.05 may be possible site signals.

- Test based on random effects model for continuous variables

  For continuous variables, such as BMI, blood pressure, baseline continuous biomarker, and medical device success rate, etc., the random effects model developed by Desmet et al. [37] can be applied to identify sites with significantly different values of mean when compared with other sites. Using a random effects model, for a continuous variable, the outcome for subject s in site i is modeled as $y_{is} = \mu + \gamma_i + e_{is}$, with $\gamma_i \sim N(0, \tau^2)$, $e_{is} \sim N(0, \sigma^2)$, where μ is the fixed effect, γ_i are the site-level random effects, and e_{is} are random errors. The sample mean for site i is then $y_{i.} = \frac{1}{n_{i.}} \sum_{s=1}^{n_{i.}} y_{is} \sim N(\mu, \tau^2 + \frac{\sigma^2}{n_{i.}})$, so that $y_{i.} - \mu \sim N(0, \tau^2 + \frac{\sigma^2}{n_{i.}})$. Let the maximum likelihood estimates (MLEs) of μ, τ^2, and σ^2 be $\hat{\mu}, \hat{\tau}^2, \hat{\sigma}^2$. The p-value of one-sided test (for $H_0 : \mu_i = \mu_0$ vs. $H_a : \mu_i > \mu_0$) for site i is calculated as $p_i = P(Z \geq \frac{y_{i.} - \hat{\mu}}{\sqrt{\hat{\tau}^2 + \frac{\hat{\sigma}^2}{n_{i.}}}})$; and the p-value of two-sided test ($H_0 : \mu_i = \mu_0$ vs. $H_a : \mu_i \neq \mu_0$) for site i is calculated as $p_i = 2 \times P(Z \geq abs(\frac{y_{i.} - \hat{\mu}}{\sqrt{\hat{\tau}^2 + \frac{\hat{\sigma}^2}{n_{i.}}}}))$.

  In situations where subject-level data are not available and only site-level summary data are provided, i.e., when for each site i , only the site size n_i , sample mean $y_{i.}$ and sample variance s_i^2 are available, other parameter estimation methods such as ANOVA approach or DerSimonian-Laird (DL) approach [34], can be used to estimate the reference distribution, and then the corresponding statistical tests for each site and variable pair can be carried out. Lastly, to control the FDR across the sites/rows in the presence of multiple comparisons (I), "Benjamini Hochberg (BH)" method [23] is performed for each variable, and the raw p-values are adjusted.

10.7.2 Simulation of P-values for site signals

- Significance level

  Significance level is the magnitude of p-values for individual significant test. Specifically, an example of tests with different significance levels is shown in Table 10.2, a p-value matrix with 6 study sites and 4 variables/tests. Among the 6 sites, 2 sites have significant variables/tests (Site 1 and Site 3). A variable/test is considered significant if $p_{ij} < 0.05$. Site 1 has two significant tests and Site 3 has only one significant test. Also, the observed significance level of the tests is very strong for cell (3,2) with p_{ij} equals to 0.0001, and is marginal for cell (1,1) and (1,3) with p_{ij} close to 0.05. This difference in magnitude of p-values for individual tests may have an effect on model performance.

- Generation of p-values for site signals

  We first randomly select the significant variable/tests for one site signal. As shown in Table 10.2, suppose we select Site 1 as a site with randomly selected two significant variable/tests, i.e., Var1 and Var3 for this dataset, among the total 4 variables/tests. We then simulate p-values of selected variables/tests from a pre-specified range of values for significant tests (i.e., $[0, 0.05)$ for mild significance level, $[0, 0.025)$ for moderate significance level, or $[0, 0.01)$ for strong significance level).

TABLE 10.2
Example of p-value matrix.

Site ID	Var 1	Var 2	Var 3	Var 4
1	0.048	0.8	0.045	0.5
2	0.1	0.7	0.2	0.1
3	0.2	0.0001	0.3	1
		...		
6	0.7	0.5	0.6	0.1

10.7.3 Simulation study for correlation P-values

- Fisher combination approach adjusted for correlated p-values

  The derivation of the Fisher combination approach adjusted for correlated p-values is shown below [19, 92]:

$$s_i = \sum_{j=1}^{J} -2log(p_{ij}), \text{ where } -2log(p_{ij}) \sim^{i.i.d.} \chi_2^2;$$

$$E(s_i) = 2J; Var(s_i) = 4J + 2\sum_{j=1}^{J}\sum_{J'<J}^{J} cov(-2log(p_{ij}), -2log(p_{ij'}))).$$

$$\text{Since} \frac{s_i}{c} \sim \chi_f^2; E(s_i) = cf; Var(s_i) = 2c^2 f$$

$$\text{Then, } c = 1 + \frac{1}{2J}\sum_{j=1}^{J}\sum_{j'<j}^{J} cov(-2log(p_{ij}), -2log(p_{ij'}); f = 2J/c$$

  On the other hand, $s_{-i} = \sum_{i' \neq i} s_{i'}$; since $\frac{s_i}{c} \sim \chi_f^2$; $\frac{s_{-i}}{c} \sim \chi^2_{f(I-1)}$, With the scale factor, c, and the degree of freedom, f, the corresponding p-values for s_i and s_{-i} under their Chi-squared distributions are calculated as $\tilde{p}_i = P(\chi_f^2 > s_i/c)$ and $\tilde{p}_{-i} = P(\chi^2_{f(I-1)} > s_{-i}/c)$. If the degrees of freedom for a Chi-squared is large, a normal approximation can be used to calculate these probabilities.

- Simulation results

  In this chapter, we perform a comprehensive examination of the effect of experimental conditions on the characteristics of the models. We conduct a simulation study reflecting patterns in small dataset (with small numbers of sites and tests) from PMAs for diagnostic devices. Specifically, we assume each site has 20 tests, with p-values of significant tests being simulated from $U[0, 0.01)$. Furthermore, the number of sites I in a dataset is sometimes below 20, and a dataset may contain multiple site signals, with some site signals being relatively stronger than the others. For each scenario, the correlated p-value matrix is simulated as follows:

1. Simulate x_{ij} from a multivariate normal distribution with mean =0 and a pre-set correlation structure, with half of the tests($J = 10$) highly correlated by pair-wise $\rho = 0.7$ and the other half of the tests ($J = 10$) uncorrelated. The cumulative probability of each x_{ij} under normal distribution, i.e., $p_{ij} = F(x_{ij})$, is calculated to serve as the baseline entry in p-value matrix.
2. Generate p-values for the significant variables/tests within each site signal (Appendix 10.7.2) The simulated correlated p-value matrix is analyzed by two Fisher combination approaches, one without correlation adjustment (the original version) and the other with correlation adjustment (the extended one). The result is shown in Table 10.3. Note that the results in each row in the following table are based on 1,000 simulations.

TABLE 10.3
Fisher combination approach simulation result.

		Fisher combination				Fisher combination adjusted for correlated p-values			
# of sites	# of site signals (% of significant tests per site signal	pseudo-sen	sen	spec	FDR	pseudo-sen	sen	spec	FDR
5	1 (30%)	0.93	0.91	0.97	0.08	0.93	0.76	0.99	0.03
10	1(30%)	0.89	0.96	0.96	0.17	0.88	0.63	0.99	0.07
10	2 (each with 30%)	0.91	0.74	0.98	0.08	0.91	0.24	0.99	0.04
10	3 (one with 30%, two with 50%)	0.96	0.68	1.00	0.01	0.96	0.66	0.99	0.02
10	4 (two with 30%, two with 50%)	0.97	0.43	1.00	0.00	0.97	0.60	0.98	0.02
15	1 (30%)	0.83	0.96	0.96	0.29	0.79	0.49	0.99	0.11
15	2 (each with 30%)	0.88	0.83	0.98	0.13	0.88	0.22	0.99	0.06
15	3 (one with 30%, two with 50%)	0.93	0.74	1.00	0.02	0.94	0.67	0.98	0.06
15	5 (one with 20%, one with 30%, two with 50% and one with 60%)	0.91	0.48	1.00	0.00	0.92	0.84	0.80	0.18

Table 10.3 shows that for most cases, the extended Fisher combination approach, adjusted for correlated p-values, has a lower sensitivity and a stricter control of false discovery rate, indicating that it is more conservative than the original Fisher combination approach. The advantage of correlation adjustment is seen when there are over 30% site signals in a dataset (rows 5 and 9 in Table 10.2). Finally, although the extended Fisher combination approach may be more conservative in terms of the final p-values scores when compared against its original version, both approaches share similar pseudo-sensitivities, suggesting that they can produce similar site rankings.

10.8 Tables and Figures

TABLE 10.4
Original p-value matrix based on J variables/tests and I sites.

	var 1	$\cdots$	var j	$\cdots$	var J
site 1	p_{11}	$\cdots$	p_{1j}	$\cdots$	p_{1J}
			$\cdots$		
site i	p_{i1}	$\cdots$	p_{ij}	$\cdots$	p_{iJ}
			$\cdots$		
site I	p_{I1}	$\cdots$	p_{Ij}	$\cdots$	p_{IJ}

TABLE 10.5
Dichotomized p-value matrix.

	var 1	$\cdots$	var j	$\cdots$	var J
site 1	c_{11}	$\cdots$	c_{1j}	$\cdots$	c_{1J}
			$\cdots$		
site i	c_{i1}	$\cdots$	c_{ij}	$\cdots$	c_{iJ}
			$\cdots$		
site I	c_{I1}	$\cdots$	c_{Ij}	$\cdots$	c_{IJ}

TABLE 10.6
Count table for LRT.

	# of significant vars/tests	total # of vars/tests
Site 1	n_1	P_1
		$\cdots$
Site i	$n_i = \sum_{j=1}^{J} c_{ij}$	$P_i =$ # of vars/tests with $c_{ij} \in 0, 1$, for site i
		$\cdots$
Site I	n_I	P_I
Total	$n_.$	P

TABLE 10.7
Analysis result for the case study.

Site ID	# of subs by site	Var1	Var2	Var3	Var4	...	Var17	Var18	Var19	Var20	p-value1	p-value2
1	28	1.0000	1.0000	1.0000	1.0000	...	1.0000	1.0000	0.9160	0.4620	1.0000	0.9839
2	56	0.0830	1.0000	1.0000	0.9870	...	1.0000	1.0000	1.0000	0.7880	1.0000	0.9825
3	197	1.0000	1.0000	0.0380	1.0000	...	0.0010	1.0000	0.6120	0.5500	0.7986	0.9709
4	203	1.0000	0.9980	0.9230	1.0000	...	0.9800	1.0000	0.0330	0.6050	1.0000	0.9817
5	108	0.0020	1.0000	1.0000	1.0000	...	0.9260	1.0000	0.3030	0.4180	1.0000	0.9769
6	82	1.0000	1.0000	1.0000	1.0000	...	1.0000	0.3000	1.0000	0.4650	1.0000	0.9833
7	179	0.0000	0.8880	1.0000	0.0000	...	1.0000	0.0000	1.0000	0.0020	0.0356	0.0024
8	129	1.0000	1.0000	1.0000	1.0000	...	1.0000	1.0000	0.0000	0.7110	1.0000	0.9095
9	92	0.6250	0.9720	0.3340	1.0000	...	0.0020	1.0000	1.0000	0.7090	1.0000	0.9765
10	235	1.0000	1.0000	1.0000	1.0000	...	1.0000	1.0000	0.0010	0.7980	1.0000	0.9793
11	79	1.0000	1.0000	1.0000	1.0000	...	1.0000	0.2870	1.0000	0.3240	1.0000	0.9829
13	84	0.0000	0.0460	1.0000	1.0000	...	1.0000	0.0030	1.0000	0.1010	0.0356	0.3653
14	15	1.0000	1.0000	1.0000	1.0000	...	0.9640	0.9960	1.0000	0.4680	1.0000	0.9839
15	21	1.0000	1.0000	0.2290	1.0000	...	1.0000	1.0000	1.0000	0.7520	1.0000	0.9834
17	13	1.0000	1.0000	1.0000	1.0000	...	1.0000	1.0000	1.0000	0.7650	1.0000	0.9841
18	25	1.0000	1.0000	1.0000	1.0000	...	1.0000	0.9680	1.0000	0.8820	1.0000	0.9841

pvalue1 is the overall p-value by LRT approach with thred=0.1, and pvalue2 is overall p-value by Fisher combination approach.

TABLE 10.8
Simulation setting.

# of sites (rows)	$I = 10, 20, 40, 50$
# of tests for each site (column)	$j = 10, 20, 50, 100$
p_{ij}	$U[0, 1]$
# of simulations	$N_{sim} = 10,000$

TABLE 10.9
Type-I error.

	LRT (thred = 0.1) number of tests/columns J				Fisher combination number of tests/columns J			
number of sites/rows I	10	20	50	100	10	20	50	100
10	0.008	0.0122	0.0179	0.0195	0.0801	0.084	0.0788	0.0719
20	0.0063	0.0111	0.0152	0.0182	0.072	0.0756	0.0748	0.0713
40	0.007	0.0084	0.0136	0.0164	0.0683	0.0668	0.067	0.0644
50	0.0066	0.0075	0.0126	0.0153	0.0711	0.0627	0.0662	0.0642

TABLE 10.10
Default settings.

# of sites I	40
# of tests J	50
# of site signals	1, 2, 5
% of significant tests for each site signal	20%=10 tests
p-values of significant tests	$[0, 0.025)$
N_{sim}	1,000

TABLE 10.11
Performance with different numbers of sites (I).

			LRT (thred = 0.1)				Fisher combination			
# of site signals	# of sites (I)	% of site signals	pseudo-sen	sen	spec	FDR	pseudo-sen	sen	spec	FDR
1	20	5%	0.9930	0.6430	0.9997	0.0040	0.9980	0.9820	0.9988	0.0107
2	40	5%	0.9790	0.4590	0.9998	0.0038	0.9970	0.9370	0.9997	0.0042
1	10	10%	0.9960	0.6830	0.9997	0.0015	1.0000	0.9870	0.9987	0.0060
2	20	10%	0.9875	0.4880	0.9997	0.0028	0.9975	0.9165	0.9997	0.0028
5	50	10%	0.9838	0.2814	1.0000	0.0000	0.9956	0.6586	1.0000	0.0002
1	5	20%	0.9980	0.6930	1.0000	0.0000	0.9990	0.9810	1.0000	0.0000
2	10	20%	0.9970	0.4190	1.0000	0.0000	0.9980	0.8720	1.0000	0.0000
5	25	20%	0.9924	0.1802	1.0000	0.0000	0.9974	0.4180	1.0000	0.0000
8	40	20%	0.9900	0.1206	1.0000	0.0000	0.9970	0.1759	1.0000	0.0000

sen is sensitivity and spec is specificity.

TABLE 10.12
Performance with different numbers of tests per site (J).

		LRT (thred = 0.1)				Fisher combination			
# of site signals	# of tests per site (J)	pseudo-sen	sen	spec	FDR	pseudo-sen	sen	spec	FDR
1	10	0.4300	0.0060	0.9998	0.0060	0.4000	0.0710	0.9988	0.0460
1	20	0.6820	0.0410	0.9998	0.0080	0.7700	0.3530	0.9989	0.0380
1	40	0.9380	0.3410	0.9997	0.0090	0.9780	0.8680	0.9992	0.0187
1	50	0.9810	0.5520	0.9998	0.0050	0.9980	0.9670	0.9991	0.0172
1	100	1.0000	0.9960	0.9997	0.0060	1.0000	1.0000	0.9994	0.0112
2	10	0.5765	0.0060	0.9999	0.0030	0.5210	0.0715	0.9993	0.0255
2	20	0.7650	0.0370	0.9998	0.0060	0.8090	0.2990	0.9991	0.0283
2	40	0.9555	0.2605	0.9999	0.0020	0.9845	0.8105	0.9994	0.0093
2	50	0.9855	0.4735	1.0000	0.0005	0.9940	0.9235	0.9997	0.0038
2	100	0.9995	0.9805	0.9999	0.0007	1.0000	1.0000	0.9998	0.0023
5	10	0.8106	0.0018	0.9999	0.0020	0.6738	0.0222	0.9999	0.0030
5	20	0.8610	0.0118	1.0000	0.0000	0.8666	0.1120	0.9999	0.0023
5	40	0.9686	0.1294	1.0000	0.0000	0.9830	0.4280	0.9999	0.0013
5	50	0.9894	0.2734	1.0000	0.0000	0.9954	0.6086	1.0000	0.0000
5	100	1.0000	0.9184	0.9999	0.0003	1.0000	0.9716	1.0000	0.0000

sen is sensitivity and spec is specificity.

TABLE 10.13
Performance with different percentages of significant tests per site signal.

		LRT (thred = 0.1)				Fisher combination			
# of site signals	% of significant tests per site signal	pseudo-sen	sen	spec	FDR	pseudo-sen	sen	spec	FDR
1	10%	0.5140	0.0310	0.9998	0.0080	0.5850	0.2220	0.9988	0.0400
1	12%	0.6580	0.0750	0.9996	0.0150	0.7680	0.3830	0.9990	0.0307
1	16%	0.8850	0.2330	0.9997	0.0100	0.9490	0.7580	0.9992	0.0215
1	20%	0.9780	0.5490	0.9998	0.0055	0.9950	0.9650	0.9993	0.0145
1	30%	1.0000	0.9990	0.9998	0.0030	1.0000	1.0000	0.9994	0.0120
2	10%	0.5780	0.0220	0.9998	0.0055	0.6610	0.1675	0.9991	0.0293
2	12%	0.7055	0.0480	0.9999	0.0045	0.7815	0.3090	0.9993	0.0187
2	16%	0.8955	0.1875	0.9998	0.0070	0.9460	0.6765	0.9992	0.0143
2	20%	0.9820	0.4965	0.9999	0.0015	0.9950	0.9330	0.9995	0.0067
2	30%	1.0000	0.9995	0.9999	0.0017	1.0000	1.0000	0.9999	0.0013
5	10%	0.7596	0.0148	0.9999	0.0020	0.7676	0.0940	0.9998	0.0060
5	12%	0.8110	0.0308	0.9999	0.0045	0.8476	0.1600	0.9999	0.0008
5	16%	0.9328	0.1052	1.0000	0.0000	0.9624	0.3660	0.9999	0.0018
5	20%	0.9864	0.2588	1.0000	0.0005	0.9956	0.5884	1.0000	0.0003
5	30%	1.0000	0.9188	1.0000	0.0000	1.0000	0.9676	1.0000	0.0000

sen is sensitivity and spec is specificity.

TABLE 10.14
Performance with different significance levels.

		LRT (thred = 0.1)				Fisher combination			
# of site signals	significance level	pseudo-sen	sen	spec	FDR	pseudo-sen	sen	spec	FDR
1	0.05	0.9760	0.5500	0.9998	0.0060	0.9630	0.7970	0.9991	0.0215
1	0.025	0.9840	0.5790	0.9998	0.0065	0.9940	0.9700	0.9990	0.0205
1	0.01	0.9770	0.5290	0.9998	0.0050	0.9990	0.9990	0.9995	0.0105
2	0.05	0.9820	0.4695	0.9999	0.0008	0.9605	0.7095	0.9994	0.0092
2	0.025	0.9815	0.4655	0.9999	0.0012	0.9950	0.9185	0.9995	0.0068
2	0.01	0.9810	0.4820	0.9999	0.0020	1.0000	0.9960	0.9997	0.0033
5	0.05	0.9860	0.2498	0.9999	0.0013	0.9658	0.3904	0.9999	0.0015
5	0.025	0.9854	0.2566	1.0000	0.0000	0.9960	0.6014	1.0000	0.0000
5	0.01	0.9878	0.2576	0.9999	0.0008	1.0000	0.8200	1.0000	0.0000

sen is sensitivity and spec is specificity.

Bibliography

[1] DAEN. https://www.tga.gov.au/database-adverse-event-notifications-daen.

[2] Data Extraction and Longitudinal Trend Analysis (DELTA) Registry: https://nestcc.org/portfolio-item/icd-registry-delta-active-surveillance-pilot-study/.

[3] EudraVigilance. https://www.ema.europa.eu/en/human-regulatory/research-development/pharmacovigilance/eudravigilance.

[4] FAERS. https://www.fda.gov/drugs/surveillance/questions-and-answers- fdas-adverse-event-reporting-system-faers.

[5] https://www.nih.gov/health-information/nih-clinical-research-trials-you/list-registries.

[6] Kaiser Permanente National Implant Registries. https://national-implantregistries.kaiserpermanente.org/.

[7] MAUDE. https://www.accessdata.fda.gov/scripts/cdrh/cfdocs/cfmaude/search.cfm.

[8] MEDSUN. https://www.accessdata.fda.gov/scripts/cdrh/cfdocs/medsun/searchreporttext.cfm.

[9] MHRA. https://aic.mhra.gov.uk/era/pdr.nsf/Search?openform.

[10] NEISS. https://www.cpsc.gov/Research–Statistics/NEISS-Injury-Data.

[11] Vigibase. https://www.who.int/medicines/news/glob_pharmvig_database_qa/en/.

[12] What is a serious adverse event? available from https://www.fda.gov/safety/reporting-serious-problems-fda/what-serious-adverse-event.

[13] U.S. Food and Drug Administration. *Guidance for Industry: Good Pharmacovigilance Practices and Pharmacoepidemiologic Assessment.* https://www.fda.gov/media/71546/download, 2005.

[14] European Medicines Agency. *Guideline on the Use of Statistical Signal Detection Methods in the Eudravigilance Data Analysis System.* http://www.ema.europa.eu/ docs/en_GB/document_library/ Regulatory_and_procedural_guideline/ 2009/11/WC500011434.pdf, 2008.

[15] A. Agresti. *Categorical Data Analysis (Second edition).* John Wiley & Sons, Ltd, NEW Jersey, 2002.

[16] I. Ahmed, C. Dalmasso, F. Haramburu, F. Thiessard, P. Broët, and P. Tubert-Bitter. False discovery rate estimation for frequentist pharmacovigilance signal detection methods. *Biometrics*, 66(1):301–309, 2010.

[17] I. Ahmed, F. Haramburu, A. Fourrier-Reglat, F. Thiessard, C. Kreft-Jais, G. Miremont-Salame, B. Gegaud, and P. Tubert-Bitter. Bayesian pharmacovigilance signal detection methods revisited in a multiple comparison setting. *Statistics in Medicine*, 28:1774–1792, 2009.

[18] K. Ahrar and S. Gupta. Hepatic artery embolization for hepatocellular carcinoma: technique, patient selection, and outcomes. *Surgical Oncology Clinics of North America*, 12(1):105–126, 2003.

[19] G. Alves and Y-K. Yu. Accuracy evaluation of the unified p-value from combining correlated p-values. *PLOS One*, 9(3):e91225, 2014.

[20] D. Banks, E.J. Woo, D.R. Burwen, P. Perucci, M.M. Braun, and R. Ball. Comparing data mining methods on the VAERS database. *Pharmacoepidemiology and Drug Safety*, 14:601–609, 2005.

[21] D. Basu and R. Tiwari. A note on the Dirichlet process. *Statistics and Probability: Essays in Honor of C. R. Rao. New York: North-Holland*, pages 89–103, 1982.

[22] A. Bate, M. Lindquist, and I.R. Edwards. A Bayesian neural network method for adverse drug reaction signal generation. *European Journal of Clinical Pharmacology*, 54(4):315–321, 1998.

[23] Y. Benjamini and Y. Hochberg. Controlling the false discovery rate: a practical and powerful approach to multiple testing. *Journal of the Royal Statistical Society Series B (Methodological)*, 50(1):289–300, 1995.

[24] D. Blackwell and JB. MacQueen. Ferguson distributions via polya urn schemes. *The Annals of Statistics*, 1(2):353–355, 1973.

[25] M. Borenstein, L.V. Hedges, J.P.T. Higgins, and H.R. Rothstein. *Introduction to meta-analysis.* John Wiley & Sons, Ltd, 2009.

[26] A. Briasoulis, C. Inampudi, E. Akintoye, O. Adegbala, P. Alvarez, and J. Bhama. Trends in utilization, mortality, major complications, and

cost after left ventricular assist device implantation in the united states (2009 to 2014). *The American Journal of Cardiology*, 121(10):1214–1218, 2018.

[27] J.S. Brown, M. Kulldorff, K.R. Petronis, R. Reynolds, K.A. Chan, R.L. Davis, D. Graham, S.E. Andrade, M.A. Raebel, L. Herrinton, D. Roblin, D. Boudreau, D. Smith, J.H. Gursitz, M.J. Gunter, and R. Platt. Early adverse drug event signal detection within population-based health networks using sequential methods: key methodologic considerations. *Pharmacoepidemiology and Drug Safety*, 18(3):226–34, 2009.

[28] Center for Devices and Radiological Health. U.S. Food and Drug Administration webpage. `https://www.fda.gov/medical-devices/products-and-medical-procedures/obesity-treatment-devices`.

[29] D.R. Challoner. Medical devices and the public's health: the FDA 510(k) clearance process at 35 years. *Written Statement before the Committee on Health, Education, Labor, and Pensions US Senate, Institute of Medicine of the National Academics, Washington*, 2011.

[30] C.R. Charig, D.R. Webb, S.R. Payne, and J.E. Wickham. Comparison of treatment of renal calculi by open surgery, percutaneous nephrolithotomy, and extracorporeal shockwave lithotripsy. *British Medical Journal (Clinical Research ed.)*, 292:879, 1986.

[31] L.X. Clegg, E.J. Feuer, D.N. Midthune, M.P. Fay, and B.F. Hankey. Impact of reporting delay and reporting error on cancer incidence rates and trends. *Journal of the National Cancer Institute*, 94:1537–45, 2002.

[32] A.J. Cook, R. Tiwari, R.D. Wellman, S.R. Heckbert, L. Li, P. Heagerty, T. Marsh, and J.C. Nelson. Statistical approaches to group sequential monitoring of postmarket safety surveillance data: Current state of the art for use in the mini-sentinel pilot. *Pharmacoepidemiol Drug Safety*, 21:72–81, 2012.

[33] W.E. Dager, R. Gosselin, R. Raschke, and T. Vanderveen. Heparin: Improving treatment and reducing risk of harm clinical, laboratory and safety challenges. *Patient Safety & Quality Healthcare*, pages 20–25, Jan 2009.

[34] R. DerSimonian and N. Laird. Meta-analysis in clinical trials. *Controlled Clinical Trials*, 7(3):177–188, 1986.

[35] G. Deshpande, V. Gogolak, and S.W. Smith. Data mining in drug safety: Review of published threshold criteria for defining signals of disproportionate reporting. *Pharmaceutical Medicine*, 24(1):37–43, 2007.

[36] L. Desmet, D. Venet, and E. Doffagne. Use of the beta-binomial model for central statistical monitoring of multicenter clinical trials. *Statistics in Biopharmaceutical Research*, 9(1):1–11, 2017.

[37] L. Desmet, D. Venet, E. Doffagne, C. Timmermans, T. Burzykowski, C. Legrand, and M. Buyse. Linear mixed-effects models for central statistical monitoring of multicenter clinical trials. *Statistics in Medicine*, 33(30):5265–79, 2014.

[38] Y. Ding, M. Markatuo, and R. Ball. An evaluation of statistical approaches to postmarketing surveillance. *Statistics in Medicine*, 39:845–874, 2020.

[39] S.N. Doost, L. Zhong, and Y.S. Morsi. Ventricular assist devices: Current state and challenges. *Journal of Medical Devices*, 11(4):663–668, 2017.

[40] L. Duczmal and R. Assunçao. A simulated annealing strategy for the detection of arbitrarily shaped spatial clusters. *Computational Statistics & Data Analysis*, 45(2):269–286, 2004.

[41] W. DuMouchel. Bayesian data mining in large frequency tables, with an application to the FDA spontaneous reporting system. *The American Statistician*, 53(3):177–190, 1999.

[42] W. DuMouchel and D. Pregibon. Empirical Bayes screening for multi-item associations. *KDD*, pages 67–76, 2001.

[43] M. Dwass. Modified randomization tests for nonparametric hypotheses. *Annals of Mathematical Statistics*, 28:181–187, 1957.

[44] L. Ensign and K. Cohen. A primer to the structure, content and linkage of the FDA's manufacturer and user facility device experience (MAUDE) files. *The Journal for Electronic Health Data and Methods*, 5(1):12, 2017.

[45] S.J. Evans, P.C. Waller, and S. Davis. Use of proportional reporting ratios (PRRS) for signal generation from spontaneous adverse drug reaction reports. *Pharmacoepidemiology and Drug Safety*, 10(6):483–486, 2001.

[46] FDA Bioresearch monitoring program Website: https://www.fda.gov/MedicalDevices/DeviceRegulationandGuidance/ Overview/Bioresearch Monitoring/default.htm.

[47] R.A. Fisher. *Statistical Methods for Research Workers.* Oliver & Boyd (Edinburgh), 1925.

[48] U.S. Food and Drug Administration. *Strengthening Our National System for Medical Device Postmarket Surveillance: Update and Next Steps.* https://www.fda.gov/media/84409/download, 2013.

[49] U.S. Food and Drug Administration. *Serious adverse events with implantable left ventricular assist devices (LVADs): FDA Safety Communication.* U.S. Food and Drug Administration, Silver Spring, MD, 2015.

[50] U.S. Food and Drug Administration. *Factors to Consider Regarding Benefit Risk in Medical Device Product Availability, Compliance, and Enforcement Decisions: Guidance for Industry and Food and Drug Administration Staff.* U.S. Food and Drug Administration, Silver Spring, MD, 2016.

[51] U.S. Food and Drug Administration. *Best Practices in Drug and Biological Product Postmarket Safety Surveillance for FDA Staff.* U.S. Food and Drug Administration, Silver Spring, MD, 2019.

[52] U.S. Food and Drug Administration. *Center for Devices and Radiological Health. Medical Device Databases.* https://www.fda.gov/medical-devices/device-advice-comprehensive-regulatory-assistance/medical-device-databases., 2019.

[53] U.S. Food and Drug Administration. *FDA-Approved Devices That Keep the Heart Beating.* https://www.fda.gov/consumers/consumer-updates/fda-approved-devices-keep-heart-beating, 2019.

[54] S.N. Forjuoh, J.W. Helduser, J.N. Bolin, and M.G. Ory. Challenges associated with multi-institutional multi-site clinical trial collaborations: Lessons from a diabetes self-management interventions study in primary care. *Journal of Clinical Trials*, 5(3):219, 2015.

[55] J.M. Gibbons, G.M. Cox, A.T.A. Wood, J. Craigon, S.J. Ramsden, D. Tarsitano, and N.M.J. Crout. Applying Bayesian model averaging to mechanistic models: an example and comparison of methods. *Environmental Modelling and Software*, 23:973–985, 2008.

[56] G.N. NorSAn G.N., A. Bate, and R. Orre. Extending the methods used to screen the who drug safety database towards analysis of complex associations and improved accuracy for rare events. *Statistics in Medicine*, 25(21):3740–3757, 2006.

[57] M. Goodman, Y. Li, and R. Tiwari. Detecting multiple change points in piecewise constant hazard functions. *Journal of Applied Statistics*, 38:2523–2532, 2011.

[58] S. Gottlieb. Reflections on a landmark year for medical product innovation and public health advances and looking ahead to policy in 2018. *FDA Voice*, 2018.

[59] S. Gottlieb and J. Shuren. New steps to facilitate beneficial medical device innovation. *FDA Voice*, 2018.

[60] D. Grady. *Breast Implants Linked to Rare Cancer Are Recalled Worldwide.* The New York Times. https://www.nytimes.com/2019/07/24/health/breast-implants-cancer-recall.html, 2019.

[61] P.E. Greenwood and M.S. Nikulin. *A Guide to Chi-Squared Testing.* Wiley, New York, 1996.

[62] T.M. Gross, B.W. Bode, D. Einhorn, D.M. Kayne, J.H. Reed, N.H. White, and J.J. Mastrototaro. Performance evaluation of the minimed® continuous glucose monitoring system during patient home use. *Diabetes Technology & Therapeutics*, 2(1):49–56, May 2000.

[63] IMDRF Adverse Event Terminology Working Group. *IMDRF Terminologies for Categorized Adverse Event Reporting (AER): Terms, Terminology Structure and Codes.* The International Medical Device Regulators Forum, 2020.

[64] Y.S. Guan, Y. Hu, and Y. Liu. Multidetector-row computed tomography in the management of hepatocellular carcinoma with transcatheter arterial chemoembolization. *Journal of Gastroenterology and Hepatology*, 21(6):160–167, 2006.

[65] D.B. Hall. Zero-inflated Poisson and binomial regression with random effects: A case study. *Biometrics*, 56:1030–1039, 2000.

[66] J. Hartung, G. Knapp, and B.K. Sinha. *Statistical Meta-analysis with Applications.* John Wiley & Sons, Ltd, 2011.

[67] M. Hauben and J. K. Aronon. Defining 'signal' and its subtypes in pharamcovigilance based on a systematic review of previous definitions. *Drug Safety*, 32(2):99–110, 2009.

[68] M. Hauben, S. Horn, and L. Reich. Potential use of data-mining algorithms for the detection of 'surprise'. *Drug Safety*, 30(2):143–155, 2007.

[69] M. Hauben, D. Madigan, C.M. Gerrits, L. Walsh, and E.P.V. & Puijenbroek. The role of data mining in pharmacovigilance. *Expert Opinion on Drug Safety*, 4(5):929–948, 2005.

[70] M. Hauben, L. Reich, Micco J. De, and K. Kim. Extreme duplication in the US FDA adverse events reporting system data base. *Drug Safety*, 30(6):551–554, 2007.

[71] R.G. Hauser, A.S. Mugglin, P.A. Friedman, D.B. Kramer, L. Kallinen, D. McGriff, and D.L. Hayes. Early detection of an underperforming implantable cardiovascular device using an automated safety surveillance tool. *Circulation: Cardiovascular Quality and Outcomes*, 5(2):189–196, 2012.

[72] A.M. Hochberg, S.J. Reisinger, and P.K. Pearson. Using data mining to predict safety actions from FDA adverse event reporting system data. *Drug Information Journal*, 41:633–644, 2007.

[73] L.V. Holle and V. Bauchau. The upper bound to the relative reporting ratio—a measure of the impact of the violation of hidden assumptions underlying some disproportionality methods used in signal detection. *Pharmacoepidemiology and Drug Safety*, 23:787–794, 2014.

[74] N. Hu, L. Huang, and R. Tiwari. Signal detection in FDA AERS database using Dirichlet process. *Statistics in Medicine*, 34:2725–2742, 2015.

[75] T. Hu, L. Huang, J. Xu, and R. Tiwari. Spatial-cluster signal detection in medical devices using likelihood ratio test method. *Therapeutic Innovation & Regulatory Science (TIRS)*, 55:56–64, June 2020.

[76] T. Hu, J. Xu, L. Huang, Z. Xu, Z. Yao, and R. Tiwari. Likelihood ratio test method for multiple medical device comparison using multiple site safety and effectiveness data with continuous outcomes. *Therapeutic Innovation & Regulatory Science (TIRS)*, 54(6):1444–1452, Nov 2020.

[77] L. Huang, T. Guo, J. Zalkikar, and R. Tiwari. A review of statistical methods for safety surveillance. *Therapeutic Innovation & Regulatory Science*, 48(1):98–108, 2014.

[78] L. Huang, R. Tiwari, Z. Zou, M. Kulldorff, and E.J. Feuer. Weighted normal spatial scan statistic for heterogeneous population data. *Journal of the American Statistical Association*, 104(487):886–898, 2009.

[79] L. Huang, J. Zakikar, and R. Tiwari. Likelihood ratio test based method for signal detection in drug classes using FDA's AERS database. *Journal of Biopharmaceutical Statistics*, 23:178–200, 2013.

[80] L. Huang, J. Zalkikar, and R. Tiwari. A likelihood ratio test based method for signal detection with application to FDA's drug safety data. *Journal of the American Statistical Association*, 106(496):1230–1241, April 2011.

[81] L. Huang, J. Zalkikar, and R. Tiwari. Likelihood ratio based tests for longitudinal drug safety data. *Statistics in Medicine*, 33:2408–2424, 2014.

[82] L. Huang, J. Zalkikar, and R. Tiwari. Likelihood-ratio-test methods for drug safety signal detection from multiple clinical datasets. *Computational and Mathematical Methods in Medicine*, 2019.

[83] L. Huang, D. Zheng, J. Zalkikar, and R. Tiwari. Zero-inflated Poisson model based likelihood ratio test for drug safety signal detection. *Statistical Methods in Medical Research*, 26(1):471–488, 2017.

[84] C. Jennison and B.W. Turnbull. *Group Sequential Methods with Applications to Clinical Trials*. Chapman & Hall/CRC New York, 2000.

[85] A.S. Julious and M.A. Mullee. Confounding and Simpson's paradox. *BMJ*, 309:1480–1481, 1994.

[86] M.Y. Jung, R. Ward, Z. Xu, J. Xu, Z. Yao, L. Huang, and R. Tiwari. Application of a likelihood ratio test based method for safety signal detection to left ventricular assist devices. *Journal of Biopharmaceutical Statistics*, pages 1–8, June 2020.

[87] K. Katsanos, S. Spiliopoulos, P. Kitrou, M. Krokidis, and D. Karnabatidis. Risk of death following application of paclitaxel-coated balloons and stents in the femoropopliteal artery of the leg: A systematic review and meta-analysis of randomized controlled trials. *Journal of the American Heart Association*, 7(24), 2018.

[88] H. Khalili, E.S. Huang, B.C. Jacobson, C.A. Camargo, D. Feskanich, and A.T. Chan. Use of proton pump inhibitors and risk of hip fracture in relation to dietary and lifestyle factors: a prospective cohort study. *British Medical Journal*, 344:e372, 2012.

[89] A. Kirisits and W.K. Redekop. The economic evaluation of medical devices. *Applied Health Economics and Health Policy*, 11(1):15–26, 2013.

[90] E. Kontopantelis and D. Reeves. Performance of statistical methods for meta-analysis when true study effects are non-normally distributed: A simulation study. *Statistical Methods in Medical Research*, 21(4):409–426, 2012.

[91] E. Kontopantelis, D.A. Springate, and D. Reeves. A re-analysis of the cochrane library data: The dangers of unobserved heterogeneity in meta-analyses. *PLoS ONE*, 8(7):e69930, July 2013.

[92] J.T. Kost and M.P. McDermott. Combining dependent p-values. *Statistics & Probability Letters*, 60(2):183–190, 2002.

[93] B.M. Kuehn. Heparin: Improving treatment and reducing risk of harm clinical, laboratory and safety challenges. *Journal of the American Medical Association*, 299(12):1417, 2008.

[94] M. Kulldorff. A spatial scan statistic. *Communications in Statistics - Theory and Methods*, 26(6):1481–1496, 1997.

[95] M. Kulldorff, I. Dashevsky, T.R. Avery, A.K. Chan, R.L. Davis, D. Graham, R. Platt, S.E. Andrade, D. Boudreau, M.J. Gunter, L.J. Herrinton, P.A. Pawloski, M.A. Raebel, D. Roblin, and J.S. Brown. Drug safety data mining with a tree-based scan statistic. *Pharmacoepidemiology and Drug Safety*, 22:517–523, 2013.

[96] M. Kulldorff, R.L. Davis, M. Kolczak, E. Lewis, T. Lieu, and R. Platt. A maximized sequential probability ratio test for drug and vaccine safety

surveillance. *Sequential Analysis: Design Methods and Applications*, 30:58–78, 2012.

[97] M. Kulldorff, Z. Fang, and S.J. Walsh. A tree-based scan statistic for database disease surveillance. *Biometrics*, 59:323–331, 2003.

[98] M. Kulldorff, L. Huang, L. Pickle, and L. Duczmal. An elliptic spatial scan statistic. *Statistics in Medicine*, 25(22):3929–3943, 2006.

[99] S. D. Lalonde, A.C. Alba, A. Rigobon, H.J. Ross, D.H. Delgado, F. Billia, M. McDonald, R.J. Cusimano, T.M. Yau, and V. Rao. Clinical differences between continuous flow ventricular assist devices: A comparison between HeartMate II and HeartWare HVAD. *Journal of Cardiac Surgery*, 28(5):604–610, 2013.

[100] D. Lambert. Zero-inflated Poisson regression, with an application to defects in manufacturing. *Technometrics*, 34:1–14, 1992.

[101] K.K.G. Lan and D.L. Demets. Discrete sequential boundaries for clinical trials. *Biometrika*, 70:659–663, 1983.

[102] L. Li. A conditional sequential sampling procedure for drug safety surveillance. *Statistics in Medicine*, 28:3124–3138, 2009.

[103] Y. Liang and P. Zhao. Similarity search in graph databases: a multi-layered indexing approach. In: *2017 IEEE 33rd International Conference on Data Engineering (ICDE)*, 2017.

[104] T.A. Lieu, M. Kulldorff, R.L. Davis, E.M. Levis, E. Weintraub, K. Yih, R. Yin, J.S. Brong, and R. Platt. Real-time vaccine safety data surveillance. *Medical Care*, 45(2):S89–95, 2007.

[105] D Madigan, A Genkin, DD Lewis, and D. Fradkin. Bayesian multinomial logistic regression for author identification. In *Proceedings of the 25th International Workshop on Bayesian inference and Maximum Entropy Methods in Science and Engineering (MaxEnt 05)*, pages 509–516, 2005.

[106] D. Madigan, P. Ryan, S. Simpson, and I. Zorych. Bayesian methods in pharmacovigilance. *Bayesian Statistics 9*, pages 421–438, 2011.

[107] Medical Device Reporting (MDR). Available from https://www.fda.gov/medicaldevices/safety/reportaproblem/.

[108] D.N. Midthune, M.P. Fay, L.X. Clegg, and E.J. Feuer. Modeling reporting delays and reporting corrections in cancer registry data. *Journal of the American Statistical Association*, 100(469):61–70, 2005.

[109] L.W. Miller and J.G. Rogers. Evolution of left ventricular assist device therapy for advanced heart failure: A review. *JAMA Cardiology*, 3(7):650–658, 2018.

[110] E.J. Molina and S.W. Boyce. Current status of left ventricular assist device technology. seminars in thoracic and cardiovascular surgery. *JAMA Cardiology*, 25(1):56–63, 2013.

[111] L.H. Monsein. Primer on medical device regulation. part i. history and background. *Radiology*, 205(1):1–9, 2013.

[112] K. Nam, N.C. Henderson, P. Rohan, E.J. Woo, and E. Russek-Cohen. Logistic regression likelihood ratio test analysis for detecting signals of adverse events in postmarket safety surveillance. *Journal of Biopharmaceutical Statistics*, 27(6):990–1008, 2017.

[113] S.E. Nissen and K. Wolski. Effect of rosiglitazone on the risk of myocardial infarction and death from cardiovascular causes. *New England Journal of Medicine*, 356:2457–2471, 2007.

[114] G.N. Noren, J. Hopstadius, A. Bate, K. Star, and I.R. Edwards. Temporal pattern discovery in longitudinal electronic patient records. *Data Min Knowl Disc*, 20:361–387, 2010.

[115] G.N. Noren, R. Sundberg, A. Bate, and I.R. Edwards. A statistical methodology for drug-drug interaction surveillance. *Statistics in Medicine*, 17(16):3057–70, 2008.

[116] G.N. Norén, A. Bate, R. Orre, and I.R. Edwards. Extending the methods used to screen the who drug safety database towards analysis of complex associations and improved accuracy for rare events. *Statistics in Medicine*, 25(21):3740–3757, 2006.

[117] P.C. O'Brien and T.R. Fleming. A multiple testing procedure for clinical trials. *Biometrics*, 35:549–556, 1979.

[118] P. Palatini, G. Frigo, O. Bertolo, E. Roman, R. Da, and M. Winnicki. Validation of the a&d tm-2430 device for ambulatory blood pressure monitoring and evaluation of performance according to subjects' characteristics. *Blood Pressure Monitoring*, 3(4):255–260, August 1998.

[119] A. Pariente, F. Gregoire, A. Fourrier-Reglat, and F.N.M. Haramburu. Impact of safety alerts on measures of disproportionality in spontaneous reporting databases: the notoriety bias. *Drug Safety*, 30(10):891–8, 2007.

[120] J. Pearl. *Probabilistic Reasoning in Intelligent Systems: Networks of Plausible Inference.* Morgan Kaufmann, San Mateo, CA, 1988.

[121] Platt, R. and Carnahan, R. The U.S. Food and Drug Administration's Mini-Sentinel Program. Available from https://onlinelibrary.wiley.com/doi/pdf/10.1002/pds.3230.

[122] A. Prinzing, U. Herold, A. Berkefeld, M. Krane, R. Lange, and B. Voss. Left ventricular assist devices—current state and perspectives. *Journal of Thoracic Disease*, 8(8):660, 2016.

[123] J. G. Rogers, F.D. Pagani, A.J. Tatooles, G. Bhat, M.S. Slaughter, E.J. Birks, S.W. Boyce, S.S. Najjar, V. Jeevanandam, and A.S. Anderson. Intrapericardial left ventricular assist device for advanced heart failure. *New England Journal of Medicine*, 376(5):451–460, 2017.

[124] K.J. Rothman, S. Lanes, and S.T. Sack. The reporting odds ratio and its advantages over the proportional reporting ratio. *Pharmacoepidemiology and Drug Safety*, 13(8):519–523, 2004.

[125] E. Roux, F. Thiessard, A. Fourrier, B. Begaud, and P. Tubert-Bitter. Evaluation of statistical association measures for the automatic signal generation in pharmacovigilance. *IEEE Transactions on Information Technology in Biomedicine*, 9(4):518–527, 2005.

[126] P. Sajgalik, A. Grupper, B.S. Edwards, S.S. Kushwaha, J.M. Stulak, D.L. Joyce, R. Joyce, C. Daly, T. Kara, and J.A. Schirger. Current status of left ventricular assist device therapy. *New England Journal of Medicine*, 91(7):927–940, 2016.

[127] T. Sato. Hepatic artery embolization for hepatocellular carcinoma: technique, patient selection, and outcomes. *Seminars in Oncology*, 29(2):160–167, 2002.

[128] M.J. Schuemie. Methods for drug safety signal detection in longitudinal observational databases: LGPS and LEOPARD. *Pharmacoepidemiology and Drug Safety*, 20(3):292–299, 2011.

[129] J. Sethuraman. A constructive definition of Dirichlet priors. *Statistica Sinica*, 4:639–650, 1994.

[130] J. Sethuraman and R. Tiwari. Convergence of Dirichlet measure and the interpretation of their parameters. *Statistical Decisions Theory and Related Topics III*, 2:305–315, 1982.

[131] R. Starling, N. Moazami, S.C. Silvestry, G. Ewald, J.G. Rogers, C.A. Milano, J.E. Rame, M.A. Acker, E.H. Blackstone, and J. Ehrlinger. Unexpected abrupt increase in left ventricular assist device thrombosis. *New England Journal of Medicine*, 370(1):33–40, 2014.

[132] Surveillance, Epidemiology, and End Results Program (SEER). https://seer.cancer.gov/. Accessed October 7, 2019.

[133] A. Szarfman, S.G. Machado, and R.T. ONeill. Use of screening algorithms and computer systems to efficiently signal higher-than-expected combinations of drugs and events in the us FDA's spontaneous reports database. *Drug safety*, 25(6):381–392, 2002.

[134] U.S. Food and Drug Administration. Device Approvals-HeartWare HVAD, Available from https://www.fda.gov/medicaldevices/productsandmedicalprocedures/DeviceApprovalsandClearances/RecentlyApprovedDevices/ucm581473.htm.

[135] U.S. Food and Drug Administration. Premarket Approval (PMA), https://www.accessdata.fda.gov/scripts/cdrh/cfdocs/cfpma/pma.cfm. Accessed July 29, 2019.

[136] R. Voelker. New standards reduce heparin potency. *Journal of the American Medical Association*, 302(18):1956, 2009.

[137] L.A. Waller and C.A. Gotway. *Applied Spatial Statistics for Public Heath Data*. Wiley Hoboken, NJ, USA, 2004.

[138] S.V. Wang, J. Maro, E. Baro, R. Izem, I. Dashevsky, J. Rogers, M. Nguyen, J. Gagne, E Patorno, K. Huybrechts, J. Major, E. Zhou, M. Reidy, A. Cosgrove, S. Schneeweiss, and M. Kulldorff. Data mining for adverse drug events with a propensity score-matched tree-based scan statistic. *Pharmacoepidemiology*, 29:895–903, 2013.

[139] R.L. Wardrop. Simpson's paradox and the hot hand in basketball. *The American Statistician*, 49(1):24–28, 1995.

[140] E.J. Woo, R. Ball, D.R. Burwen, and M.M. Braun. Effects of stratification on data mining in the us vaccine adverse event reporting system (VAERS). *Drugs Safety*, 31(8):667–674, 2008.

[141] C.F.J. Wu. On convergence properties of the EM algorithm. *Annals of Statistics*, 11:95–103, 1983.

[142] J. Xu, L. Huang, Z. Yao, Z. Xu, J. Zalkikar, and R. Tiwari. Statistical methods for clinical study site selection. *Therapeutic Innovation & Regulatory Science*, 54(1):211–219, 2020.

[143] Z. Xu, T. Kass-Hout, C. Anderson-Smits, and Gray G. Signal detection using change point analysis in postmarket surveillance. *Pharmacoepidemiology and Drug Safety*, 26(6):663–668, 2015.

[144] Z. Xu, J. Xu, Z. Yao, L. Huang, M. Jung, and R. Tiwari. Evaluating medical device adverse event signals using a likelihood ratio test method. *Journal of Biopharmaceutical Statistics*, pages 1–10, June 2020.

[145] Y.X. Yang, J.D. Lewis, S. Epstein, and D.C. Metz. Long term proton pump inhibitor therapy and risk of hip fracture. *Journal of the American Medical Association*, 296(24):2947–2953, 2006.

[146] F. Yates. Contingency table involving small numbers and the x2 test. *Journal of the Royal Statistical Society*, 1(2):217–235, 1934.

[147] G.V. Yule and M.G. Kendall. *An Introduction to the Theory of Statistics.* Charles Griffin, London, 1957.

[148] X. Zhao, C. Xiao, X. Lin, Q. Liu, and W. Zhang. A partition-based approach to structure similarity search. *Proceedings of the VLDB Endowment*, 7(3):169–180, 2013.

[149] Y. Zhao, M. Yi, and R. Tiwari. Extended likelihood ratio test-based method for signal detection in a drug class with application to FDA's adverse event reporting system database. *Statistical Methods in Medical Research*, pages 1–15, 2016.

[150] I. Zorych, D. Madigan, P. Ryan, and A. Bate. Disproportionality methods for pharmacovigilance in longitudinal observational databases. *Statistical Methods in Medical Research*, 22(1):39–56, 2013.

Subject Index

Printed in the United States
by Baker & Taylor Publisher Services